UNDERSTANDING STROKE

For patients, carers and
health professionals

NEW REVISED EDITION

by
ROSEMARY SASSOON
with contributions by
specialists in the field

Book Guild Publishing
Sussex, England

This edition published in Great Britain in 2013 by
The Book Guild Ltd
Pavilion View
19 New Road
Brighton, BN1 1UF

First edition published in the UK in 2002 by
Pardoe Blacker Publishing Limited

Typesetting in Minion by
Keyboard Services, Luton, Bedfordshire

Printed in Great Britain by
CPI Antony Rowe

A catalogue record for this book is available from
The British Library

ISBN 978 1 84624 843 6

Rosemary Sassoon has had a varied working life, first as designer and letterer, then as a researcher, writer and lecturer specialising in the educational and medical aspects of handwriting. This study included all ages from pre-school children to adult neurological patients. It was this work that first introduced her to the problems of stroke patients. The University of Reading awarded her a PhD for her work on children's handwriting. More recently she researched and designed a family of typefaces specially for educational purposes. She lectures and researches worldwide on handwriting and letterforms and is author of some fifteen books. Having a stroke has not stopped her.

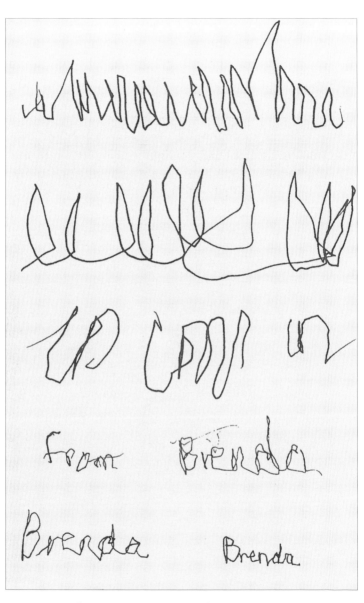

The stages in retraining a stroke patient to write.

Contents

Part 3

Part 4

Preface to Second Edition

THE FIRST EDITION of *Understanding Stroke* was published ten years ago and by now needed to be updated and extended. This book looks at stroke from different perspectives – it provides the patient with the information and motivation so vital for successful rehabilitation. It has helped carers to understand many of the issues involved, and at the same time it bridges the gap between patients and health professionals, who have benefited from a clearer picture of the problems from the patient's point of view.

In the second edition my own part is much extended, however, I have left the original section unaltered. It is the perception of an informed patient (I had been involved in some areas of neurorehab research long before my own stroke) two years post stroke. As such it is just as relevant as ever to anyone concerned with that stage of recovery. What I have done, however, is to expand the end of this section.

In the past decade I have learned a lot more – from my own experiences, from what other patients have confided, from responses to presentations I have made as well as learning from other speakers and research literature. Although I do not want to make this too much of a personal account, inevitably this part is written from the perspective of a long-term (and somewhat elderly) stroke survivor. This is an aspect that is not often considered, and deserves more thought. There are many thousands of us.

The issues that concerned me then still concern me: the level of information for patients and carers and even for some doctors, communication with patients in hospital, especially those suffering from aphasia, and the lack of understanding of how to motivate people to help their recovery. Surely the understanding of stroke and stroke care itself has much improved in the last decade, both of prevention and after-care, but reports from around the country still seem to vary enormously. Some parts of the country have excellent services, but not all.

Other contributors have added to their sections, though not all when they considered that their contributions were still relevant and adequate. There is a new chapter entirely, contributed by Tom Balchin, founder of the ARNI Trust, concerned with specific areas of rehabilitation. Professor Alan Wing and his group at Birmingham University have provided a completely new chapter on research. It not only deals with taking part in neurorehabilitation research, but also, with such matters as psychology and neurorehabilitation, and gives a thorough, yet easily comprehensible explanation of neuro-plasticity. His team also gives a recent example of their research.

The Stroke Association has updated their section listing new research, websites and contacts. As with the first edition, I expect them to review and recommend it on their list, as do the Scottish Heart and Stroke Association, Different Strokes and other stroke groups with which I have been associated.

We all hope that this new edition will continue to be of use to patients, carers and health professionals, as it has been in the past.

Introduction

RESEARCHING FOR THIS BOOK has made me realise how little I knew when I suffered my stroke and how much I would have liked to have such information myself when it was most necessary. In many cases, and in the first instance, it will be partners, parents or carers who might need to absorb and pass on the information included here, and the philosophy of hope and self-help that is propounded in the first part. But this book has a dual purpose, which will become clear as the reader progresses.

Patients need to understand their own condition and the role of the different health professionals they will encounter during their rehabilitation, and those nurses, therapists and even doctors need to understand more about the feelings and effects of the condition on their patients. This book is meant to be as relevant to them as to those they are treating. A successful outcome depends as much on a victory over the mind as over the body. I hope this will help to change some of the entrenched attitudes on the subject that hold back both patients' and professionals' expectations.

Many books about stroke suffer because the writers have not experienced a stroke themselves. They may be factually correct and useful but lack the insight that could bring them to life. Then there are those that are solely a personal report, enthralling and sometimes uplifting to read, but as strokes are so different in the way that they affect individuals, these may not be entirely relevant to patient, carer or health professional. It is hard to judge what is relevant to a reader in such a diverse subject. Patients' intelligence should not be underestimated. They and their carers deserve the highest level of information. Health professionals also would profit from as wide a perspective as possible on their patients' needs.

The first edition of this book evolved over a period of four years. It was two years after my stroke before I felt I had a balanced enough perspective of what had happened to record my observations. Over the next two years colleagues with whom I have worked in the past, alongside those who I had met during my recovery, have contributed their sections. As a result the contents of the book were and still are divided between a personal report and some valuable professional perspectives. Although the range is wide, the concerns of every aspect of patient care cannot be fully discussed. It should, however, awaken readers to the many possibilities (and some of the problems) concerned with rehabilitation.

Nothing I have heard in the intervening year from other patients, their carers, and parents of young children, or read during my recovery, has changed my view. Care and provision of information are regrettably patchy and often unsatisfactory. In a report from the Stroke Association, *Speaking Out About Stroke Services* (June 2001) one of the surveys indicated the particular need to meet the requirements of patients with psychological and psychiatric problems as a result of stroke. In that report one patient was reported as saying: 'Hospital staff should be made more aware of the variety of problems resulting from stroke. Sadly most disregard the feelings of patients and some even make fun of the situation'.

What happens in a crowded, understaffed geriatric ward is very different from the ideal put forward by the trainers of today's therapists. My feedback from patients all around the country has been about the lack of facilities and understanding of individual needs. Nothing that I have reported has been exaggerated, though I have concentrated on the National Health Service and not investigated private health care where undoubtably excellent care is obtainable in some places for those who can afford it.

You only need to read the informative publications from Different Strokes to understand that the plight of young stroke sufferers is even less addressed than that of the elderly. The situation of child stroke patients is no better understood. From those I come into contact with through my work in education, where their medical needs may, with luck, be adequately dealt with, their educational and psychological needs are seldom comprehended, much less met.

Much thought and planning is taking place at present into provision for the care of stroke patients. It still may take many years before enough young therapists and specialist nurses are trained – and more consultants and specialist doctors. With them will come the new attitudes towards their patients – because it is attitudes that need changing. That is just as important as more resources.

Acknowledgements

M Y THANKS must first go to all the contributors: to friends I have worked with in the past, to those who contributed so much to my recovery and those I have met since – or have not yet had the pleasure of meeting. (The part they all played is explained in the book.) They are all busy professionals who have written their chapters in the cause of disseminating knowledge to stroke survivors and their carers and sharing it with other health professionals. I owe a lot to many people in the various organisations, especially the Stroke Association, who patiently answered my queries and provided me with vital information. I think that I can safely say that there will be many readers who will also owe thanks to them.

I would like to thank Elwyn Blacker as well as his wife Jeanne Blacker. As both editor and publisher Elwyn encouraged me to complete this somewhat unconventional multi-level book – when others doubted if it could work.

I would like to dedicate this book to my husband John, without whose loving care I would not have been able to make such a good recovery.

Part 1

FROM THE
PATIENT'S PERSPECTIVE

1
Before

FEW PEOPLE are lucky enough to have had any specialised knowledge to prepare them for the experience of a sudden stroke. I was fortunate. Some years ago I took part in a project at the suggestion of Alan Wing who was then at the Medical Research Council Applied Psychology Unit, Cambridge. He is now Professor of Human Movement at Birmingham University. It concerned those who had lost the use of their natural writing hand – the educational and medical aspects of handwriting being my special interest at that time. It was intended to concentrate on the problems of directionality involved in having to use the non-preferred hand. Stroke patients came into that category as well as others suffering neurological impairment. The work was never published, but it served me very well in the end as it brought me into contact for the first time with those recovering from a stroke and those who cared for them. This project seemed a logical extension of my work with complex handwriting problems, but soon showed that there were some unexpected benefits from using handwriting to help in the retraining of a non-functional hand. A presentation of this work at an Eastern Motor Group meeting led to other contacts, and more patients. The impressions I formed then were to affect my attitude to my own recovery some fifteen years later.

Learning from patients

My small local hospital ran a stroke club about that time. It seemed a good starting place for research. The speech therapist who ran it ensured that her frail and elderly patients (mainly men) enjoyed their intensive speech therapy. There was a cheerful and positive atmosphere in the dark and dreary hut where the activities took place. It felt more like a social club than a hospital. However, in those days there were no occupational therapists working locally. I had a special interest in observing how patients were being retrained to write, but found that this was left to volunteer helpers – ladylike, caring but totally unskilled. Patients were encouraged to learn to write with their non-preferred, undamaged hand. Nothing was being done to help retrain their natural writing hand. They were being taught to use capital letters in the misguided assumption that they would find it easier. In fact, the constant repositioning of the pen required in the writing of capital letters is usually much more difficult for anyone getting used to their non-preferred hand. This also applies to anyone with a tremor, from whatever cause. It should be recommended only when the writer previously wrote solely in capital letters.

Case 1 taught me how some patients found their own solutions, even in the face of inappropriate advice. This also made me consider that it might actually be counter-productive to encourage the use of the non-preferred hand except when absolutely essential. The gradual return to the use of the right hand, in a way that was visible and could be monitored, would signal progress towards normality and might have an even deeper meaning to a patient.

An elderly man, who had suffered a stroke some two years before, was proudly presented as the group's most successful patient. He was indeed managing to write a passable script with his left hand. When asked if he had ever tried to write with his right hand the answer was: 'Of course I can write perfectly well now with my right hand but I haven't told the kind ladies here because they seem so pleased that they have taught me to use my left hand'. There seemed no understanding of the value of retraining his right (preferred) hand.

The patient's left-handed *(above)* and right-handed writing *(below)*.

That man recounted something that many patients have mentioned since, that he did not feel that his left-handed writing was really a true representation of himself, and he only felt comfortable once he could return to his old writing, however shaky it was at first.

Case 2 gave me an opportunity to investigate how to use handwriting to be a visible and welcome sign of progress for patients themselves. The idea of using handwriting as an aid to diagnosis is far from original. This patient showed that the written trace could be a useful measure for health professionals to monitor returning motor function, and other aspects of a patient's condition. It showed unexpected additional benefits in countering depression and helped me to formulate my ideas about the effects of motivation on a patient's attitude to recovery.

It was the usual practice then to delay therapy for several weeks, so it was not easy to gain access to patients to assess the effect of early intervention. However, in a nearby nursing home, was a woman in her mid-forties who had just suffered her second stroke. A teacher, she despaired of ever returning to her profession. To show her that she would be able to write again seemed a first step towards regaining her confidence. There were no facilities at the hospital, so we borrowed a piece of hardboard and rested it at an angle against the bed as she sat by it. The patient was encouraged to make any mark she could with a felt pen, supporting her (considerably) damaged right hand with her left, in any way that was comfortable.

The illustration on the frontispiece shows how it is quite easy to make any stroke (in the graphic sense of the word) into the resemblance of some letter or other. In two or three sessions, over a period of about three weeks, this lady progressed to a passable signature – one of the most important things for any disabled person to acquire. It is the way you present yourself to the world. Without a signature, even with the advent of computers, you are forever dependent on someone else to deal with your business affairs if you are unable to fill in a form, or sign a cheque.

The therapists and nurses involved in this patient's care expressed astonishment at her progress. 'She could suddenly begin to use a knife and fork', said one. 'She even managed to open a window', said another the next week. It transpired that the only exercises that she would have been offered to improve hand function would have been to have two boxes and told to practise transferring buttons from one to another. This was hardly inspiring or motivating to an intelligent and distressed patient. Practising and watching the gradual improvement of your own script is quite another matter. The woman, with little else to do, was constantly striving to improve her signature, and in doing so made great strides in improving her hand function. What this did for her self-confidence and relief from depression was evident to us all.

Case 3 has considerable implications for those who despair because they have lost the ability to communicate, and for those who care for them. The point to make here is that because the power of speech is temporarily (or even permanently) impaired there is no reason to assume that the ability to write has been affected. It is always worth trying to see if the patient is still able to communicate through writing.

It was some years later, in Singapore, when a physiotherapist invited me to join her on her rounds. She wanted me to see a distinguished Chinese patient who did not seem to be making the progress that she had expected. She described how he had been an eminent public figure and had always dreaded becoming disabled and unable to communicate. In the position he now found himself, his worst fears had been realised. He lay motionless on the bed, not even trying to co-operate with the physiotherapist. I asked his nurse if he had been offered any kind of indicator board to help him to have some small degree of control, perhaps choice over his food or drink. The reply was that the hospital could not afford such luxuries, and I had to point out tactfully that all I meant was a piece of paper with some simple drawings on it.

I found myself asking if anyone had ever tried to find out whether the patient could write with his functional hand. This provoked an uproar, and some most unfortunate remarks by the nurse about the patient's mental state that, in her considered opinion, would preclude any such activity. One look at the patient's eyes made us realise that we had made a breakthrough. A piece of paper and a pencil were grudgingly found and the patient produced a perfect sequence of Chinese characters with his left hand. I never found out what he had written because none of us could read Chinese, but I heard later that, though confined to a wheelchair, the patient otherwise made a full recovery.

Case 4 illustrated the consequences of what can occur when appropriate treatment is not available. Strokes are not confined to the elderly, far from it. One young stroke patient, a boy of about nine years old, was brought to me by his teacher who was worried that he had problems trying to write with his left hand. It appeared that he had had very successful therapy for his right leg at a London teaching hospital, and no longer showed any signs of a limp. He was supposed to have had therapy for his arm after he returned home. For whatever reason, this had not taken place. He held his right arm behind him. He said it was his enemy, and that the children at school called him the one-armed bandit.

It seemed to me that there was no reason why he should not be able to retrain his right hand, and get it functional. I was only going to see him once so there was little time to find out. I sat him at the kitchen table and put a packet of chocolate biscuits in front of him and told him that he could take the first one with his left hand but then he must use his right one if he wanted any more. It was fascinating to watch him. His hand seemed to go through all the stages of development, but gradually he controlled the contortions, and by the end of the packet was quite efficient. It was then a short step to show him that he was perfectly capable of holding a pencil in his right hand, and with practise, he should be able to begin to write. But it was not to be. Another school year brought a change of teacher; it was later reported that, without further help or encouragement, frustration and behavioural problems set in.

Conclusions

These, and other patients helped me to formulate my ideas. Even though my area of research was specialised and somewhat limited, it seemed to me that all patients reacted positively to active motivation, especially to something with visual feedback. Encouragement roused them from their apathy and they all responded to being treated as intelligent people. It appeared that this had not always been the case. Their particular talents, their home environment and their future expectations all had to be considered. Then with practical, realistic encouragement, and the respect that everyone deserves, whatever therapy they received would be more effective. I saw evidence in some of the cases that came my way of the waste of human potential and the disastrous consequences of inadequate therapy, and depressing, ill-informed care. I was not particularly well informed about what might have been happening in major teaching hospitals and other centres of excellence, but my recent personal experiences and observations have not led me to change my mind.

My interest then shifted, to dystonia patients, investigating the problems of writer's cramp patients at several London hospitals over a period of five years. I had to acquire a little basic neurology, and during that time attended a few seminars and presentations – and occasionally gave them – but that was all the knowledge I brought with me to inform me when, somewhat ironically, I suffered a stroke one day after my sixty-seventh birthday.

2
Observations as a patient in hospital

THE STROKE ASSOCIATION carried out an exhaustive survey in 1999 entitled: *Stroke Care – A Matter of Chance*. It reported that: 'More people suffering from strokes are now getting progressive and co-ordinated stroke care. But the most striking results show clearly the haphazard nature of access to this care… If patients do not have access to such care they are more likely to die, and if they survive are more likely to be disabled.' The *Daily Telegraph*'s article *There is Life after Stroke* (13 April 1999) discussed this report, and again highlighted unacceptable regional variations, as well as delays and inadequacies that result in thousands of avoidable deaths and more disabilities for those who survive. It is not only articles like this, which went on to chronicle individual patients' experiences, but confirmation from many other sources that convinced me that my experiences and observations were not exceptional. I am not interested in implying criticism of hard-pressed National Health hospitals, but in analysing my impressions of how it felt to be a patient in such a way that it might be of interest or use to others.

The overriding need for all patients is to be informed and reassured – to understand what has happened to them and what is the likely outcome. It must be a terrifying experience to regain consciousness in a hospital, unable to move, unable to speak and with no understanding of what has occurred. From what I witnessed myself in hospital, the most unfortunate patients were those unable, even temporarily, to communicate. This is how one man explained what happened to him when he had a stroke in his late twenties: when he regained consciousness in a busy south London hospital he could neither move, speak or swallow. People talked about him, and over him in terms he could not comprehend. When, after about three days, he heard a doctor say that they could do no more for him, and to call an ambulance, he was quite convinced that he was going to be sent home to die. Needless to say he was being transferred to a rehabilitation unit and subsequently made a full recovery. Many years later he could still recall his anguish, and it upset him to talk about it. I was lucky, my stroke started slowly, I recognised what was happening even before I saw a doctor, and knew approximately what to expect – though, perhaps just as well, I had little idea of how long my recovery would take.

Motivation

The next imperative is for everyone involved in the care of patients to put as positive a slant as possible on everything, to provide encouragement and motivation. For most patients recovery is going to be a battle. If this is called a challenge then the emphasis is slightly altered. The sooner it is explained that the more you help yourself the better the outcome will be, the benefits of any therapy will be compounded. To be involved in your own recovery and be given partial responsibility for its success gives impetus, then every action becomes therapy. What you find difficult is what you can aim to improve. I do not want to make this chapter too much of a personal account, but some aspects may be of general interest.

Although I could not record my first impressions at the time, they are still vivid. My right side was completely paralysed, other than a little movement in my fingers. Patients had, in the past, described to me the feeling when their bodies refused to obey the dictate of their brain, but to experience it is another matter. The terms 'neural plasticity' or 'the forging of new pathways' are often discussed and I knew my brain had to find new ways of producing a movement now the part that used to control that function was damaged. The normal channels did not work so I tried to 'think' my wrist to move. The way I would describe it is that at first there was no contact between me and my wrist. Amazingly, there was soon a quiver. I cannot remember how many days it was before I could raise my hand an inch from the bed, but the connection was made and only needed to be strengthened. I had a goal now, and the motivation to reinforce this quiver.

The term 'brain damage' has frightening connotations for the general public. Changing the term 'stroke' to 'brain attack', as is being suggested, may not make the matter much better. Patients need to understand their condition. That would be the first step towards motivating them to help themselves. Maybe it would be difficult for other than a neurologist to convey to stroke patients the wonderful capacity of our brain to reorganise, and not everyone would be able to comprehend. It is asking a lot, but a simple explanation might be a comfort and an encouragement to those for whom it seemed appropriate. Families also would benefit from a bit of hope in those early, distressing days.

Depression and tiredness

I recall an incongruous episode some time during my first few days in hospital. A pleasant young man in a white coat, perhaps a medical student, appeared at my bedside. He was carrying a clipboard and almost his first question was 'On a scale of 1 to 10 how depressed did I feel?' When I replied that I did not feel at all depressed this confused him as if there was no space to record an answer like that. Many, if not most, patients are depressed to some degree, and who can blame them. Apart from the shock of what they are experiencing at that moment, and their worries about the future, most people's perception of the results of a stroke are coloured by memories of an elderly, disabled, infirm relative. I witnessed some patients who were deeply troubled, and the over-worked nursing staff had little time to counsel them. Medication is obviously needed at the deeper levels of depression. However, I gained the impression that much could be done to alleviate some of the very genuine worries of these patients with a little thought. Someone could take the time to explain as simply and clearly as possible what was going to be done to help the patient and what they could do to help themselves. Even when the patient appears uncomprehending this is important. This is surely part of the training of all concerned nowadays, but in the rush and realities of a crowded ward it seems, from many people's experience, that this does not take place.

To complicate the issue, most stroke patients would agree that tiredness becomes a fact of life, in hospital and long after. Tiredness and lethargy can be confused with depression. You can fight it, moan about it or recognise the benefits sleep brings. You may be retraining every action that you once took for granted: your speech, of course, also the way you laugh, the way you yawn or sigh. Trying to dress is tiring, and any kind of therapy even more so. Visitors are tiring and often interrupt those times when you would be better resting, and letting your body assimilate what you have learned in therapy sessions.

Early intervention

When I had been doing my earlier work it had still been the policy to delay rehabilitation for a considerable time. I had formed a strong conviction that early intervention was desirable, if only to reassure patients. In the interest of describing good practice, this is what occurred that first morning, when, in a non-specialist ward, I asked to see a physiotherapist. The neuro-physiotherapist who appeared sized up the situation and drew some graphic diagrams in green felt pen. These she fixed above my bed to show every passing nurse how to straighten my limbs. The strategically placed pillows she recommended made a huge difference to my comfort.

The medical staff reacted positively to her pictorial instructions and I am convinced that the very early intervention was extremely valuable. It reminded me how the Singapore physiotherapist (see page 19) had stressed that one of her main jobs was straightening the limbs of her home-based patients and trying to train their relatives to do likewise. Until we have specialist stroke units in every district hospital, nursing staff need to know such common sense techniques.

I should add here that in my particular case I did not feel that it was a disadvantage being placed in the early stages in an orthopaedic ward, as in many cases it would be. First of all I knew what to ask for and found that excellent therapist. She also dealt with those first rather frightening days, trying to achieve as much as to enable me to stand up. But it was something else entirely that was the most help in coming to terms with what had happened. Everyone else was so cheerful. The atmosphere did not allow me to dwell too much on my troubles. Only too soon I was dispatched to a geriatric rehabilitation unit where the physiotherapy was of the same excellent standard – but the atmosphere depressing, even daunting.

The benefits of helping yourself

Patients need to understand that to help themselves in any way they can is the best way forward. From the beginning it would be beneficial even if it could be stressed how just a little stretching in bed to reach objects (instead of ringing for the nurse or doing without) would help.

At the acute stage patients may have to accept help with everything. However, even to start learning to dress yourself can be presented positively as useful therapy. It does not matter how long it takes to fasten a button, or make the reluctant fingers of a non-preferred hand support the inefficiency of the damaged one, if it is all related to a gradual recovery. Learning new strategies to dress will be tiring, and time consuming, but there is plenty of time. If it is all explained as therapeutic, then, as each task becomes a little easier, self-esteem and optimism will rise.

My attitude was not only influenced by thinking of the benefit to be gained by exerting myself a little more each day, but of a deep hate of being dependent. Dignity and privacy are hard to find on a busy ward. One of the selling points of private medical care is that it ensures privacy. That appeals to many people, but it denies you the camaraderie of the public ward, and sometimes the constant observation that you get in an acute NHS ward. When it comes to an emergency, and this includes a stroke, then the shock of a public ward is reinforced by this stereotypical concept of the desirability of a private room.

There are obvious tiresomenesses and indignities as a result of not being mobile. There are plenty of wheelchairs on any ward, but I noticed that patients were not encouraged to try to make use of them. When one day I was left in a wheelchair after a therapy session I tried it out around the ward. My efforts were greeted with surprise and by the remark: 'Our ladies never try to take themselves around and only a few of our men'. Apart from the immediate benefits, if patients are going to be wheelchair dependent as soon as they are released, it might be a good idea for them to have a bit of practice first.

Eating and drinking

Serious incidents of eating and drinking problems are recognised and dealt with – but I am not so sure about marginal ones – and they do affect the patient's confidence and wellbeing. Eating, with one side of the body out of action, is never going to be easy. In hospital there seemed to be little between total assistance with feeding and none at all. Those who could not communicate were again at a disadvantage. They had no choice in the matter of food or drink and, as so often, a simple indicator chart (tea/coffee, milk/sugar) might have helped.

I now know that swallowing is a common – and sometimes a serious – problem. The Stroke Association has a leaflet concerned with swallowing problems and I wish I had had access to it when I really needed to understand what was happening to me. I found it a couple of years later on a stand at an out-patient clinic. The leaflet starts by explaining that swallowing is a very complicated process involving many muscles. If any one of these is not working properly there may be a difficulty with eating and drinking, especially when combining solids and liquids. One of the first questions I was asked on admission was whether I could swallow. I obediently gulped, and not knowing any better, replied, yes. From that day onwards I was puzzled by the fact that I could usually swallow food, yet had difficulty with liquids. Being cheerful meant that it was assumed all was well, but long after returning home I had to contend with swallowing difficulties, and found it difficult to make myself drink enough. There were alarming occurrences of choking. Two years later I still have to be careful.

Dealing with spasms and cramps

There is not necessarily much pain after a stroke. There may be frightening experiences, like choking and there is another uncomfortable problem, another of the many issues that patients deserve to have explained to them. That is a mixture of involuntary movement, spasms and cramps due, I now realise, partly to the contraction of muscles, and not being able to turn over easily during sleep. These annoyances seemed at the time quite positive indicators of returning movement as they affected, most markedly, the parts of my body that were just becoming mobile. If rationalised that way they seemed quite welcome. Other patients confirm my own experience that these cramps and spasms may continue for many months or even longer. They would benefit from help with strategies to minimise the effect, such as avoiding too much stretching or any abrupt movements, straightening limbs very slowly and in small stages. Having a hot shower on waking is also a great help.

Record keeping for the patient's sake

A brief diary, whoever keeps it, might well help both patient and a partner or family to accept what is happening. I read with some envy of Robert McCrum's efforts in keeping a diary – and not only as an aid to writing his book *My Year Off.** In the hospital where I treated most of my dystonia patients, their progress was recorded on video. This was intended for research and training purposes, but proved therapeutic for the patients. It enabled them to see how much they had improved in a short period of time. When everything still seems grim, it may be difficult for stroke patients or their families to appreciate the progress that is being made, and it would give them encouragement. Maybe this technique is used in some rehabilitation units; if not it might be worth a try.

Preparing for discharge

A stroke patient has a lot of planning to do before undertaking any new action such as getting in and out of a chair, much less a car, and there is plenty to think about before returning home. How they will manage in the outside world is a major concern for many patients. For those who need it, the occupational therapists will pay a pre-discharge visit to their homes to advise on safety and other matters. There is usually an excellent service for lending out necessary equipment, wheelchairs, bath seat, etc. A care package can deal with such matters as delivering meals if

---

*Picador 1998

necessary. In the interest of alleviating worry all this should be explained long before the patient is ready to leave.

Our hospital, in common with many, did not provide therapy sessions at the weekend. The staff were quite positive about letting those about to be discharged have a trial day at home (or even a night) beforehand. Contrary to many people's expectations, the hospital was in no hurry to discharge me. They made it quite clear by stressing that there was no time limit to my stay. My physiotherapist made it even clearer, warning me that I would be sacrificing my daily sessions for a very limited service 'outside'. Little did I know how limited it was to prove to be or I might have stayed another week or so – but it was Easter. To return after three days of freedom would not have been easy. It was the first of many issues that were to be balanced in the next few months – therapy and safety against motivation and functional improvement. In other words, would I progress more quickly at home with all the motivation to move and use my hand, free from the increasingly depressing atmosphere of what was becoming more of a general geriatric ward, with more of its share of dementia patients, than a rehabilitation unit? For those living alone or in unsuitable accommodation, the decision would have had to be different. I was deemed just about safe enough to transfer myself from chair to chair, and up the stairs, so with thanks but few regrets I was homeward bound the day before Good Friday. I had been in hospital for nearly two months.

3
At home

AFTER THE INITIAL EUPHORIA of being back in your own home, there is a realisation that quite a lot of the habits of a lifetime will have to change. Those around you may also have to adjust their lifestyles. It will take a lot of planning and involve compromises on both sides – but most of all on yours. If you set out with the idea that you are going to improve and get back your mobility and independence as soon as possible, then it is not so bad to sit back a little and give up some of your former role in the home or elsewhere. Usually common sense will prevail as it becomes obvious that you are not yet able to do many things that you once took for granted. An optimistic outlook is essential to both patients and carers, but it is not easy to find the right balance in everything. Too much assistance may stifle initiative. It may risk sapping the patients' confidence in their ability to get better, and turn them into permanent invalids. Then, when the family loses confidence in their ability to cope, there is a risk of institutionalising elderly patients. After all, it is only by attempting and practising the very actions that you find difficult that you slowly improve.

Too little assistance and the whole system may fail in a different way. The patients might also lose all confidence in the future through constant failure. They might take too many risks and be in danger of falling, or become frustrated by the sudden limitations on their life. Once again it depends on so many factors. Within a marriage or steady relationship, for instance, the challenge of changing roles can result in anything from a disaster to a deeper understanding and satisfaction. The patient's partner needs consideration too, Having to take all the responsibility of home, family, and perhaps business as well as caring, is a heavy burden for anyone.

Compromise will be needed in many things – in shopping for instance, when you suddenly become dependent on someone else. It is amazing what you can manage without, with a bit of ingenuity. You will probably have to drop your standards temporarily, in many ways such as tidiness in the home. To ignore the rampaging weeds in the garden could be just as difficult for some people, as I found myself. It will be hard not to get frustrated, but in the circumstances there is not much else to do. Positive things may be happening all the time, as gradually a way of coping becomes clearer. A certain satisfaction comes when different strategies are found for dealing with some of the jobs in the home.

The contrast between in hospital and out

Most of these factors are obvious – the comfort of having your own bed once again, being able to use the phone, choose to a certain extent your own food, go to bed when you want and get up at a sensible time of day, turn on the radio or the TV – the list is endless. There is a down side though. This is common to many other conditions, not only stroke. You feel pretty vulnerable as you realise that everything is now up to you or your family. There may no longer be someone to call if anything goes wrong, if you fall or drop something vital and find it impossible to retrieve it. Your own clumsiness becomes more evident and breakages and the messes resulting from dropped meals and spilled drinks are almost inevitable. There may even be moments of real panic when you find yourself in a position that you cannot resolve.

There will be decisions large and small that need to be taken when you would rather sleep and forget about it all. Some people will understand how you feel, some may consider you unhelpful, even wilful, and some people will try and take over matters that you would rather they left alone. Whatever the situation you will be expected to be grateful. You have to learn to receive graciously and yet are unable to give – you have to learn fast, and it is not always easy. It helps you and all concerned if you are more courteous than usual. This may seem an odd thing to say, but I at least found it made me feel better.

Safety at home

The most important issue is safety. Assuming that you will already have the basic equipment to help you become as independent as possible, the planning can begin. The balance is always between going forward and keeping up your morale, and safety. A broken bone as the result of a fall can be devastating on top of neurological impairment.

Stairs can be a risky and tiring manoeuvre but it is often possible to plan so you do not have to undertake it more than once a day and, initially, not unattended. Later on the same sort of rule could be applied to going outside – not to venture forth unless someone is within hearing distance. It is far harder for anyone on their own to take the small risks that seem essential to functional progress. 'Mother would never have got out of her chair again unless one of us went in every day and encouraged her to walk up the garden,' said one acquaintance. What motivates a person to become mobile and independent must vary considerably. It may be to be able to visit grandchildren perhaps, a desire to go to church, to do your own cooking, to return to work, or sheer determination not to be defeated. As one person put it: 'My father hated what the stroke had done to him so much that he was determined to beat it'. Everyone needs a bit of encouragement if they are going to recover. Whatever the motivation it is going to mean hard work and patience – and perhaps imagination – on the part of all concerned.

Conserving energy

There is another compromise and that affects all aspects of daily life. Energy is likely to be limited so that a judgement has to be made as to whether it is worth expending it on any particular act. It is still there as stamina improves – there is always more that needs doing or you want to do than you will be able – or other people think you should do. That is true of all life in general, but in this situation it is just more obvious, and the effects more serious.

The effects of getting overtired could last several days. Movement, speech, memory and other factors can be temporarily affected by over-tiredness. There are likely to be all kinds of helpful suggestions from friends and family – therapy, alternative and conventional, that may be available only at a distance, beneficial or socially desirable activities, etc. However, to get to them would be far too tiring and time-consuming to justify their benefits. It is always necessary to listen to your body. Only the patient can judge whether any particular activity is worth getting exhausted for. One small warning. However energy consuming it may be it is not worth ignoring regular eye and dental checkups. They can easily be overlooked in the new situation with quite serious consequences.

Then there is the matter of different times of day. Mental and physical energy will vary according to the time of day. This can be affected by medication. Some people will progress during the day and become more stretched and flexible. They feel better in the evening and find it far easier and more effective to do exercises then. Things that they would not be able to do in the mornings because of being too stiff, work better then. Other people report the opposite. It is one more factor to notice and plan for so as to get the best out of each day. Extremes of heat or cold may affect a patient recovering from a stroke much more than in the past. Any small setback, such as a minor infection, can affect your progress. To be more accurate, it may cause you to regress and it is important to understand that what is happening is only temporary and not become discouraged.

Out-patient physiotherapy

The real difference between being an in-patient and an out-patient is therapy – no more comforting daily sessions, no more expert help and encouragement. I was warned on the ward that things would not be the same, but nothing prepared me for the limited and comparatively inexpert therapy I received from that day on. I realise now that that was probably just a local problem. Where we live, even if a patient could afford a private neuro-physiotherapist there was none nearby. I knew then that it was basically up to me whether I got better or not. The same situation seems to arise all over the country, according to dozens of other people I have talked to, and the consequences for those who do not know how to help themselves must be much more serious. Away from large cities and hospitals, few people seem to get adequate therapy once they leave hospital. It may vary from trust to trust, and the situation should improve, but I can only report my experiences in an affluent area of the south-east, from 1998 onward.

The whole treatment of stroke patients after they leave hospital can be seriously inadequate. The superficial explanation is that the NHS is underfunded; but there are several more issues involved. One is the relationship between doctor and therapist. Stroke patients are usually referred to the local physiotherapy service. Appeal to the GP is still possible, but then his or her remoteness and increasing lack of expertise make the need for intervention difficult to establish and its form difficult to prescribe. Once the stroke patient has left hospital and been referred for therapy, the GP has lost effective control. The selection and training (or retraining) of therapists does not always seem to have kept pace with the enlargement of their responsibilities. Large hospitals, with their concentration of acute patients and specialist equipment need, and are a magnet for, the most able therapists. As a result the quality of out-patient therapy, particularly neurophysiotherapy, can vary widely. I suspect country areas suffer most.

Attitudes

Other people's attitudes cannot help but affect your confidence. The attitudes of your general practitioner, therapist and district nurse become important, especially to those who have no one else to share their successes or discuss their worries. If your GP is not sympathetic, you or your family should search for a replacement, because it is essential that all of you should have confidence in your medical adviser. One recovering patient raised another point. She felt insecure and inadequate when she did not conform to what she termed the 'time signposts' suggested by doctors and others. Told that she should have progressed faster she felt threatened by what she felt was being judged against vague guidelines. Again it seems important how such goals are suggested. Minor, realistic targets can be a challenge, but any targets set in a negative way – you will not be able to do this, or you cannot expect to do this for a long time – can be a real deterrent. One of the worst of these is to be told that after a certain time has passed you cannot expect further improvement. Sadly this is a common experience, and one that has to be challenged.

The attitude of friends and family can also affect the patient. Some people made it clear that they thought that the stroke was basically the end for me – the end of my working life and usefulness at least. This of course is what the general perception of a stroke patient is and in turn affects how some people react to you thereafter. It is almost the same as a bereavement. I have heard others recount how acquaintances cross over the road rather than meet them face to face because they do not know what to say. You can see it in the faces of people in shops and restaurants and occasionally overhear comments. Anyone who has used a wheelchair knows this kind of thing only too well. It also affects how others offer help. Many people are afraid of long term commitment. They would rush to visit and help a patient with a broken leg, but a stroke patient – that is an open-ended commitment, and let us be honest, most people today lead rushed lives. It is when you return home that visits from friends become so important. It is then that you could easily begin to feel isolated and lonely, especially if you live alone.

When first venturing out and about acquaintances can, inadvertently, be a real menace. You need all your attention so as not to trip on uneven surfaces. To turn round, or even look up, can be quite dangerous at that stage. Yet acquaintances rush up from all directions and ask you whatever you have done to yourself. Worse still they may insist on taking your arm, which immediately throws you off balance. Then there are the constant explanations and the look of shock and embarrassment on the faces of people who expected to hear of a broken bone or a hip replacement, and instead hear of a stroke.

Attitudes to walking aids

Aids to mobility are there to be used when essential, but it is vital not to become dependent on any one longer than strictly necessary. It is a big step to leave the safety of the wheelchair and take your first steps from living room to the kitchen, leaning on a stick. It is real progress, a significant triumph and the first judgement to make between support and safety. The next step may be for how long a leg splint may be either needed or even desirable, or built up shoes or even a stick. Ideally the decision should be taken jointly by patient and physiotherapist, but the real situation is often far from ideal. It is at such a time, as Jane

Cast (page 68) points out, that the patient is likely to be out of contact with therapists, just when they could do with sound advice and encouragement. The decision of when to stop depending on a walking aid is just as important as having advice earlier on about the availability of suitable aids. In the end the final decision will be taken by the patients in the privacy of their own home, balancing safety against a gradual return to normality. Much may once more depend on the attitude of those around them, family and friends – either encouraging them to take a calculated risk and move on, or worrying too much about safety and holding them back.

A personal note

It soon became apparent that my cheerful demeanour confused people. Some, like my hospital physiotherapists, approved of it and made use of the fact that I was not sunk in depression. Many people underestimated the severity of my disabilities, and that was reflected back on the way I thought. That was no bad thing at the time, though perhaps later on it was a bit of a disadvantage when I may have been judged as being less in need of help than I was. Then there were those who seemed annoyed by my optimism, and preferred to try and disillusion me. Whatever other people thought, I could not and would not have changed my reactions to the initial effects of the stroke. Privately, I was by no means always as cheerful as I appeared in public, and had some pretty black moments as I realised the implications. Somehow there did not seem to be any alternative but to appear cheerful and positive. I had learned long ago from visiting elderly relatives, how easy it is to deter visitors by detailing one's woes. Anyhow, to have given in to the many problems that still existed would not only have blighted my life but my husband's as well.

In retrospect, after two years, it is more annoying now that all the novelty has worn off. I may be much further along the path to recovery but, whereas I would have once accepted it, I now get more frustrated by my slowness and clumsiness, not less. Tiredness limits my activities, but I am constantly reminded of the effects of adrenalin (though suppressed by medication). When I really want to do something I often find it becomes possible to do it, though I may pay for it in tiredness the next day or so. When I suddenly find myself in a challenging situation I may find, to my surprise, that it is possible to meet that challenge. That confirms my feeling that you do not necessarily reach a plateau, you can always push yourself or be pushed further forward.

4
Progress and suggestions

THREE YEARS ON and the perspective shifts again. To the outsider there may be little improvement in my condition when they see me out of my home environment. To those who have not seen me since my stroke there is still the same reaction of shock and pity, but to me, and to those nearest to me, it is a different matter. Measured against some point – what I could do last year at the same time, or just last time I visited a certain place, it is obvious how much difference there is. I am no longer worried to go up a few steps without the support of a rail or banister. I can manage soft sand on the beach and get into the ocean (provided it is not too rough), a feat that was impossible last summer.

My foot seldom clumps up in panic at a bump in the path, and the nightly cramps improve slowly. It may be that I have more stamina rather than improved gait, or even that I am more relaxed and confident. I still need to concentrate on my walking when in unfamiliar surroundings and crowded pavements are still a bit of a problem. My arm is stronger and hand function is much improved from the days when I could grasp objects but had difficulty in releasing my grip – just like a baby. It is usage rather than any specific exercise that has accomplished this. Gadgets like an electric tin-opener and toothbrush have helped make some jobs easier. I am still a rather messy eater, but probably no one would notice other than myself these days.

There are even some positive improvements. My left hand was always pretty useless, but now I have become more ambidextrous. I used to speak too fast, now I am much slower which many people tell me is a great advantage. In the same way organisational powers have sharpened to devise strategies to utilise limited energy. So, in addition to speech, thinking and writing (by computer) have become better organised and perhaps deeper.

I have a greater understanding of the children with handwriting problems, dyspraxic and other, that I still see as part of my work in that field. I now know what it feels like to be able to write a few words slowly and moderately legibly, yet not be able to write anything fast. I can imagine how frustrating it must be to be criticised, and can say from experience that exercises might be counterproductive, causing more tension and deteriorating movement. I have experienced the puzzling phenomenum of the reversal of numbers. For quite a while a 6 came out when a 9 was called for and vice versa, and I was unable to take down a telephone number without several other inexplicable mistakes. Those are more reminders of the strange workings of the brain. Such problems sometimes solve themselves and, sadly, sometimes do not.

From reading this you may get the impression that I spend my time analysing my situation. Far from it, I am very lucky. The computer has enabled me to carry on my main occupation of writing books and articles on a variety of subjects. I even manage to do a certain amount of lecturing, and still see a procession of children (and a few adults) with literacy problems. As well as that I design typefaces that are meant for educational purposes and to be extra legible on the computer screen. Mentally, I am kept pretty busy and I cannot complain that life is dull – only sometimes rather tiring.

The minutiae of daily life, such as shopping, cooking and gardening take up rather more of my time than they would have done before the stroke, and I need more help with larger household tasks which I still find awkward. It is only leisure activities that are more limited through lack of mobility, as I no longer drive more than short distances, but that is not too much of a deprivation.

Small occurrences like catching flu, can still set me back and my limited efforts at handwriting (usually confined to addressing envelopes) demonstrate only too clearly when I am having a bad day. I have found that letting myself go too long without food is a mistake. Hunger seems to have as bad an effect on memory and movement as over-tiredness. Sudden thirst also needs attention, but that is not too difficult. It means keeping a bottle of water nearby when I am away from home.

Occasionally some part of me still reveals weakness or a need to be more flexible; then it is an interesting challenge to devise some exercise at home or in the swimming pool. It may not be what a therapist would recommend but usually works. The time scale may have changed but the truth is undeniable. Improvement is taking place all the time and shows no sign of reaching a plateau (a term I became conversant with early on in my convalescence).

Unexpected things remained problematic and there are times when I have had to force myself forwards. It was strangely difficult, for instance, to regain enough confidence to drive myself, long after I was judged capable of the task. It was all too easy to find some excuse why not to take the challenge, risk, or whatever you might call it. I am even more convinced now, than I was when this all began, that the battle for the mind of a patient – at any stage – is as vital as the battle for, or what may be seen as the emphasis on, the body. There is a compulsion to talk about all this, not only to confound those who declared that there would be a time limit on improvement, but to try and change the public perception of the condition.

Compiling this book has made me realise how much information I have accumulated in these last three years. At the same time it shows how little I knew about how certain parts of the body work or of the terminology of stroke rehabilitation. For example, at a vulnerable stage I was confronted by: 'Of course you trip and stub your toes, it is the result of drop foot'. How was I to know what drop foot was? I knew a bit about hands but legs and feet were outside my experience. The phrases that professionals use must seem common place to them but to patients they add to the confusion. Explanation and information can take away much of the fear and worry, and help you to understand what you can do to help yourself. Is it too much to ask for?

Inevitably, I wonder how much further on I would be by now if more and better therapy had been available, or whether my self-help methods have been just as successful. I have been fortunate, however, in other ways. The expertise and advice (if not actual therapy) of colleagues with whom I had worked earlier on, and people I became involved with by sheer luck, has had a profound effect on my recovery. I cannot recommend this self-help therapy unreservedly. It has had a reasonable outcome for me, has contributed to a kind of pride in my own achievement, and was essential as there was no provision for ongoing rehabilitation in my area, not even in the private sector. I have, however, met some people, just as determined as I was, who have not had such successful outcomes.

As I talk to more and more people I realise how lucky I have been not to have suffered any intellectual impairment, as so much has depended on my being able to plan any action in advance. It must be so much harder when you cannot communicate. Many others tell me that they suffer pain as a result of their stroke. Where there is residual pain after several years it seems even more reprehensible when they report that they have had no help.

Where can people obtain meaningful literature? If they go to their public library there is no guarantee that what they find will be appropriate or up to date. Jane Cast (see page 73) went to investigate what was available at her local library and was

43

unhappy to find only something over ten years old, that recommended practices that she considered out of date and inadequate. A book that would be useful is *Stroke at our Fingertips* by Dr A Rudd, P Irwin and B Penhale, published in 2000 by Class Publishing. It covers all aspects of life after stroke.

The Stroke Association, the only national charity concerned solely with stroke, has a comprehensive list of their own pamphlets and publications. Many people today would turn to the internet to find out more about stroke. There they will find a vast amount of up-to-date information. It is only necessary to remember that there is no censorship on the internet and it is prudent to check any medical suggestions with your doctor before acting on them.

Although it is vital that comprehensive information should be widely available, it must add to the frustration, even desperation, of patients and carers to read of management plans, intensive speech therapy, pain clinics or other assistance, when none is offered locally. The difference between what appears in the literature as the right way forward, and what is actually available country-wide is only too clear to many of us. With the best of intentions, I understand that it will be a long time before enough trained personnel will be available to implement the proposals that are now being put forward.

Suggestions

Strokes affect people in such different ways. I realise the limitations of my own experience and therefore the precise relevance of it to any other patient. I was too old for it to affect my career, yet young enough for me to have the energy to fight the effects. On the whole my damage was limited to motor functions, and I had the support of a caring husband. Certain general suggestions, however, can be made from the view of a patient. The best advice that I was given was offered about a month after my stroke. It came from a young, newly qualified physiotherapist. 'You will be improving for the rest of your life' she said. I was not willing to accept it at the time, with its depressing implication of my not being fully recovered for the rest of my life.

Now I look at it in a different light. A certain amount of long term damage is now obvious, and that message is a message of hope and not the opposite. To further that improvement the best advice I can think of is to consider any action that is tiring or awkward to perform as therapy. I recently met a lady who had not recovered full use of her arm after nearly five years. Isolated, without treatment, she said it was too tiring to use her right arm so she did not do so. I told her of my way of dealing with the same problem – months of struggling to hang out the washing (aided by making the arm work hard while swimming) managed to strengthen it. At first you may feel sick and dizzy with effort, later on only very tired, but it works in the end. You have to listen to your body and recognise the need to give in to weariness. Never be ashamed of having a rest in the afternoon, or even in the morning if you feel you need it (in the early days, the effort of getting dressed and eating breakfast was enough to make me want to retire to a comfortable sofa and have a short sleep). However, I am not aware that pushing yourself to the edge of tiredness from time to time in order to improve function does much harm. I only hope it was the correct advice for her.

It follows that with this attitude there is a need to ignore any suggested cut-off dates for further improvement. How often I heard 'You will make the most rapid recovery in the first few weeks', with the implication that as I was still in a wheelchair after two months the next stages would be slower and less successful. Then, after another two months – 'You can do almost all you need, you do not require any more therapy', indeed a suggestion that too much therapy was harmful. If I had believed that I might have given up trying there and then. Next, someone whose judgement I respect, when admiring how far I had progressed in the first year gave what was meant to be kindly advice – 'You cannot expect much more improvement after a year'. Further comments, equally kindly meant, express pleasure and astonishment that I am still so patently improving after three years. This would not come as a surprise if only attitudes could be more positive.

As I meet more people I hear the same story. One particular case of a young teenager worried me. He was more than eighteen months on in his recovery and had made good progress. He was determined and very brave – but worried. He had been told by his doctor not to expect any further progress after two years. He knew that he would not have adequate hand function, in particular, by the approaching deadline. It was obvious with his determination that the prognosis would be proven wrong, but what a cruel burden and unnecessary worry for a young boy and his parents. Others report being told that they will be confined to a wheelchair for life, when it has proved patently untrue.

Everyone needs hope, yet few people seem to be given the advice that the more they exert themselves the better their progress will be – and that they will continue to improve as long as they persevere. Progress may not be so dramatic later on, or so noticeable to others, but everyone should be encouraged to rejoice in how they are recovering even (or perhaps particularly) when it is happening slowly.

Finding new occupations

It is important to find interesting occupations that are within the capabilities of the person recovering. Many older people (or their relatives) have reported how distressed they were at being unable to continue with their usual leisure activities, such a sewing or other craft work. It is not only a feeling of uselessness that this engenders, but of boredom and does nothing to alleviate depression. Finding something suitable probably puts one more burden on carers and they may need to exercise considerable imagination (and perhaps tact as well).

I have developed a strategy that works for me when going through a bad patch. To motivate myself to get up and start the day, I think of a small task or pleasurable occupation that I would be capable of doing. It sounds rather trite, but it usually stops me from thinking of all the things I cannot do.

Some of the occupations in day centres seem rather patronising and unimaginative when offered to intelligent adults. Because you are physically disabled, temporarily or permanently, does not mean that your intellect has been affected. Painting by numbers might keep patients 'occupied' but if paints were available as well as plenty of bowls of flowers around, as I once witnessed, some people might have been offered the option of something freer and more challenging. I am probably being unfair, but this kind of incident makes me cringe. As a patient you are vulnerable in many different ways. A patient would be unlikely to complain about such a trivial matter as their intelligence being underestimated. It would be one more slight indignity to be borne among many worse. But such occurrences, added together, chip away at a person's spirit and self-confidence. It would, I suppose, boil down to the competence and willingness to go that one step further by an individual therapist,

The following example suggests that you never can foresee what will succeed and what unusual benefits a new activity might bring. In a book by American artist Barbara Roberts entitled *Catie Learns to Draw*, an interesting view is put forward. She maintains that, instead of trying to attempt something that the patients did expertly before the stroke, they should be encouraged to start new activities where there would be no negative comparison to make. Roberts illustrated some amazing work undertaken under her tuition by a stroke patient, who had never attempted any art work before. She used a technique where the drawing is done almost entirely without looking at the work in progress. What is more extraordinary is that she reports that Catie had a slight 'neglect' on her left side and needed constant prompting to look left. The art therapy seems to have helped her to overcome some of that aspect of her disability as well as giving her immense satisfaction and, as Roberts reports, a feeling of self-worth again.

Barbara Roberts was first and foremost an artist, not a therapist, which makes her contribution even more interesting. Since writing of Catie's case she has been drawn to helping more stroke patients, and talks of the incredible satisfaction that she has found in putting her skills to this usage. She reports two results which merit serious consideration. One is that all the patients seem to produce a very similar style of work; furthermore others who displayed a neglect of one side or the other improved after working with her technique.

An occupational therapist suggested that we need not think of art therapy solely in terms of painting. She felt that a more tangible and perhaps less threatening craft such as pottery might induce as immediate a sense of achievement, and be just as confidence-building. Moreover, the creating of a three dimensional piece, however simple, involves planning sequencing and other beneficial strategies. There is plenty of room for both points of view. However, Barbara Roberts' work reinforces my feelings that quite often people from a completely different field can use their special skills to benefit patients and make discoveries in ways that conventionally trained therapists would not, or could not attempt.

Perhaps I should mention here that I also went to art school and first worked as a designer and letterer, which is why I am particularly intertested in this aspect of therapy. I taught and wrote about those subjects before getting involved in the educational and medical aspects of handwriting. Finally, I turned to mainly research orientated work.

The late Sir Harry Secombe made a short television programme about his recovery from a stroke. There was a brief mention in it of music therapy, though more as a muscle strengthening activity for a man who had a classical operatic training than for pleasure. It carried the same implicit message as Barbara Roberts: that, at a vulnerable stage of recovery, it might not always be a good idea to allow comparisons between pre-stroke expertise and post-stroke capability. Watching this film – and noting the standard of therapy he was receiving – reminded me of my own resolution should I suffer a second stroke. I would gratefully accept any in-patient treatment provided by the National Health Service but would try to follow that up with a stay in one of the private rehabilitation facilities that give intensive integrated therapy.

I would make a special plea here for those who have lost the power to speak – those suffering from aphasia. There are many, like the patient mentioned on page 19, who are not being recognised as able to communicate but are quite capable of writing when given the opportunity. I met another such case when I was in hospital but could not intervene except by telling his wife what I had observed and hoping that someone would follow it up. Just recently I heard of a man who could neither speak coherently nor write, but managed to communicate his thoughts clearly by means of detailed drawings. An article in *The Times* on 10 July 2001 discussed the problem of aphasia. Part of its message was that there is hope and that there are several alternative ways of communication. A statement from the Connect centre in Borough, South London (website: www.connect.org.uk) reported: 'Most people who attend Connect's centre arrive hoping to to get their speech back. Mainly, however, the aim has to be to help them to make the most of other forms of communication, such as drawing, intonation, facial expression or gesture. We aim to help people to understand how their lives have changed.'

It may seem inappropriate to some patients that I should discuss sporting activities or even recreation. Richard Lockwood makes a case for this in *Recreation and Disability in Australia*: 'For people with disability (and this obviously applies to stroke patients among many others) recreation has been an elusive goal. With so much emphasis on planned rehabilitation the creativity and joy derived from participation has often been overridden by management constraints'. As for sport you only have to look at the paralympics to see what severely handi-capped athletes can achieve. I am not suggesting anything as dramatic as that. I remember seeing sports therapy in action in Beijing, where wheelchair-bound stroke patients were being encouraged to participate in basket ball games. In our district hospital's occupational therapy unit patients enjoyed playing darts, which had the added advantage of improving co-ordination and balance. Swimming has been my preferred activity, starting with all too brief sessions in a hydrotherapy pool, then other public pools and finally the ocean. Swimming was both excellent therapy and a pleasure. I am still not very elegant in the water, but then I never was before my stroke.

Finally, the computer provides a multitude of new opportunities for leisure and learning for all ages, as well as enabling a housebound patient to communicate with the outside world. I feel that there will be a gap in the market for challenging computer games for older people as more housebound adults depend on their computer to entertain, as well as to broaden their horizons. As the generation who use computers every day for work and recreation begin to form a larger part of older patients – whether affected from stroke or other conditions – they, quite rightly, will expect their needs to be addressed.

Stroke clubs and self-help groups

There is a desperate need to help alleviate the loneliness of many patients whose lives have become limited through loss of mobility. One way would be to start stroke clubs in the many districts where none are available. We became involved in trying to start such a group in our locality where the health authority no longer supports one. Such a group must take account of the needs of that specific community, so our first objective when we had found a suitable location, would be to set up an inaugural meeting, after publicising our intention as widely as possible. Something that could provide specialist advice, or even therapy would be ideal. Our priority was to identify the need, get something small started, then let it grow of its own accord. We have met with a few problems and have yet to succeed.

A self-help group can function at several levels, even where it is not able to provide any actual therapy. At the most basic it can provide a meeting place for patients to discuss their problems and exchange ideas. It can provide simple facilities for leisure, appropriate for those who attend. This might break down some of the feeling of isolation that many of those experience when recovering from a stroke. Helping with the organisation of such a group might add to patients' self-esteem and bring back meaning into lonely lives. At the same time a regular meeting might provide a valuable hour of freedom for carers – unless they would prefer to meet others in the same predicament and share some of their concerns.

The Stroke Association (www.stroke.org.uk) keeps a list of all affiliated stroke clubs, and more information can be obtained from their regional offices .

Different age groups have different needs. An example of what can be done can be seen in the activities of the organisation Different Strokes (see page 137) who have set up exercise groups for younger people around the country.

Alternatives

Whether a certain amount of out-patient therapy is available or not, helpful and sometimes unorthodox advice can often be gleaned from other people along the way. Some of the most useful tips I have had have come from unexpected sources. An elderly nun in hospital gave me the only help I received for dealing with a stiff, lopsided mouth. It was to try to whistle. It took a long time but eventually it worked. On holiday a couple of years later a nurse noticed my foot clumping on the cold stones as I tried to get into the swimming pool. 'Try clenching and unclenching your toes', she said – another exercise that seemed impossible at first, but helped in the end. About the same time, my daughter, who has been on the receiving end of some interesting alternative therapies, tried stimulating the nerve endings on my toes. These extremities were the last to respond to my attempts to make contact (see page 24). She was as surprised as I was when they responded with the quiver that, with perseverance, develops into controlled movement.

Alternative therapies such as aromatherapy, reflexology, and any of the many relaxation techniques might help. Different massages, tried out on my travels abroad, were particularly helpful, but I was never long enough in one place to discover whether they would have a lasting effect. I remember, some years ago, seeing a whole ward of patients in a rehabilitation hospital in Beijing undergoing acupuncture. Research is currently being undertaken in this country to determine how effective this treatment is (see page 61). It did not help me, but that was hardly a fair test as the practitioner admitted that she was just learning the technique. Also, acupuncture is probably most effective soon after a stroke, and I only tried it some two years later.

We are all, however, dependent on what is available locally. It seems to me that sensitive practitioners who will use their knowledge to adapt their techniques to your specific problem are just as important as the particular therapy itself. If I had to make a judgement I would think a mix of traditional and eastern therapies might be the perfect answer. All that it is sensible to say is that you should not expect miracles. You should try not to become too dependent on anything or anyone. That is the way to disillusionment and even despair when something or someone does not live up to expectations. Quite recently I heard of a patient who had pinned his hopes on a leg splint to help him walk again. When this failed he sank deeper into depression and gave up hope of ever becoming mobile.

An alternative, but not unorthodox, way of dealing with rehabilitation is what might be termed integrated therapy. This suggests that multi-disciplinary therapists, or at least those who have the skills and will to cross professional barriers, might be most successful. A pioneering private clinic that employs integrated therapy described their methods this way: 'Staff are skilled in each other's jobs to ensure patients are constantly stimulated. Physiotherapists talk to patients, speech therapists help them to move'.

Patients, once back in the community, in addition to their physical management deserve better understanding of what, for want of a better term, are their psychological needs. There needs to be informed encouragement from everyone concerned to assist individuals to maximise their recovery, whatever the local provision of therapy may be.

5
Ten years later

IT IS NOW more than ten years since I wrote the first edition of this book. I do not intend to alter anything. It is the perception of a patient two years post stroke, and as such is just as relevant as ever to anyone concerned with that stage of recovery. What I will do, however, is to add this extra chapter.

In the past decade I have learned a lot more – from my own experiences, from what other patients have confided, from responses to presentations I have made as well as learning from other speakers and research literature. Although I do not want to make this too much of a personal account, inevitably it is written from the perception of a long term stroke (and somewhat elderly) survivor. This is an aspect that is not often considered, and deserves more thought. There are many thousands of us.

The issues that concerned me then still concern me: the level of information for patients and carers and even for some doctors, communication with patients in hospital especially those suffering from aphasia and the lack of understanding of how to motivate people to help their recovery. Surely the understanding of stroke and stroke care itself has much improved in the last decade, both of prevention and after care, but reports from around the country seem still to vary enormously. Some parts of the country have excellent services, but not all.

On the positive side, a report in the *East Kent Stroke Journal* reported the case of someone who had a stroke on a cross channel ferry. It returned to port, an ambulance met them on the quayside, off to hospital where a stroke team had been alerted and awaited in time for a scan and thrombolising, and a very successful outcome. When I had my (stuttering) stroke the first thing I asked, as there was plenty of time, was the availability of thrombolising but no one had ever heard of it. In addition it was a Sunday and there was no one available to give the necessary scan.

On the other hand, not so long ago, I was contacted by that wonderful charity, Thrive, which encourages gardening for the disabled. I had written an article for them about a stroke survivor's garden containing some of my more unconventional methods of overcoming disability. Someone was in trouble. She told me her story over the phone and I hope if she reads this she will forgive me for including it. She sounded quite elderly and she lived in the West Country. As a result of a stroke her hand was fixed in a fist so tight that her nails were growing into the palm of her hand. All her doctor appeared to have said was to remark how brave she was in such adversity. That was seriously inadequate considering the situation, and unacceptable when relevant information is available.

If you write a book I suppose you must expect this kind of enquiry, and feeling that I can be helpful helps me too, but it is not really advisable to give advice like this over the phone. All I could suggest was either for her to contact Salisbury District Hospital to see if FES (Functional Electrical Stimulation, see page 81) would help, or to find a good neurologist and enquire about Botulinum treatment. She chose the latter with great success. The treatment would, of course, have to be repeated from time to time, which is not always too easy on the NHS, and she would benefit from having physiotherapy at the same time.

I cannot tell how much is being done to motivate patients, nor if specialists or nurses are communicating more with their patients. I can only tell you what happened when I addressed a conference for stroke nurses on just that subject. A wonderful woman jumped up, explaining that she specialised in what I think is called tube feeding. She explained that her team would group around a patient's bed to discuss the various possibilities, but never thought of explaining or asking for the patient's opinion even when they could communicate. She assured us that that would never happen again! Incidently, at that same meeting I heard a nutritionist talking about the need for stroke survivors to take most of their nutrition in the first half of the day before they and their muscles get tired. I had already found that eating in the evening made me uncomfortable, so stopped having supper. It was good to hear official justification for all my morning snacking but, more seriously, it underlines the need for all of us to listen to what our body is telling us.

I have heard little about advice for long term patients, often elderly, who are by then left to deal with things on their own. There is an attitude that stereotypes you as old and a stroke victim so often any symptom can be attributed to just that – sometimes with disastrous results. Seriously, stroke can mask other conditions. Several others have reported this attitude from doctors and others, but it could also apply to an individual's own perceptions, risking their ignoring something serious. In my case the effect of a new statin was not recognised, disguised perhaps by the other muscular pains that often plague stroke patients. Eventually I was alerted by a friend who had had similar problems. By that time some of the damage was irreversible. I hope that by now the medical profession is more alert to these problems, though I am not so sure, and I worry about saying too much about this as so many people with various conditions other than stroke are dependent on statins.

Undoubtedly a stroke alters your life but it need not spoil it. You need to try to develop new interests, maximising what you can do, not mourning what you can't and always trying to push yourself harder or you may slip backwards. Tiredness is inevitable, annoying, but not really harmful. You probably develop or enhance other skills to compensate for any disability. With me my organising skills seem to be stronger as I constantly try to organise my activities to save energy or deal with limited and sometimes painful mobility. Of course I can only speak from physical disability not from much cognitive deficit, except memory, but that is probably also partly age related. The effects of getting older are imperceptible and easily forgotten.

A friend, who was a stroke survivor and shared many of the same views, the late Ben de la Mare, wrote movingly about the spiritual impact, from the point of view of a minister in the Christian Church. His paper, published in 2005 in *Medical Humanities*, was entitled 'The Experience of Stroke and the Life of the Spirit'. Of more general matters he wrote: 'Stroke comes in many forms with very diverse outcomes. Doctors do not need telling this, but lay people do. For, in some encounters with those who have suffered a stroke, the condition is obvious. But, in others, because the signs are far from evident, the actual disabling effect of a stroke may well be underestimated. ... Some of the effects of stroke cannot be concealed, as when a degree of paralysis brings consequent disabilities and dependence on a wheel-chair; the same is true when there is a slurring of speech with facial disfigurement. Even though an erratic sense of balance, which follows trauma in the cerebellum, will make walking problematic, this is less evident to casual observers. Many other transient or temporary effects may be experienced; and there will often be an unpredictable pattern of recovery, much influenced by the presence or absence of will power. Stroke recovery brings with it complex, sometimes stormy moods: all in all an intriguing psychology. But stroke patients will be quick to remind you of the common characteristics: eg the loss of feeling or sensation, and tiredness. Another that should not be overlooked is an often well-concealed anger or frustration.'

He describes how, while relearning very basic skills like walking, writing and being sociable these aspects of our human make-up began to impress themselves on him as a model for describing the different facets of human make-up.

'First: We are all embodied. We hardly need telling that our physical form and our bodily functioning shape every other aspect of our being.

But secondly, we need to be reminded that we give ourselves to constant mental activity… But like the experience of our embodiment, our being absorbed in mental activity does not neccesarily bring us into contact with other people.

That brings us to a third facet in our human make-up, for we are relational creatures. Our creativity, our very humanity, thrives on our engagement with other people… Where there is no relationality, we are truly disabled.

The stroke patient, who is trying to fight back and to join some of the hurley-burley of so-called normal life, ought to be aware of these three facets of human life.'

He continued: 'Stroke patients with potential for improvement thrive on perceptible signs of progress ("Last week I walked a mile"). Equally, we are wise to fear those who talk knowingly about our impending arrival at a "plateau". Both patient and carer have to resist the very idea of a plateau; instead they must foster the ambition to go on getting better – whatever that means precisely'.

He gave a good example of the need for both physical and mental effort, by describing an interview with his neurologist when he was reporting his own enthusiasm and success in ever longer walks as therapy: The unexpected response was: 'Yes – but what end? Where is the mental stimulation?' 'He caught me on the raw, and I knew it. So, a whole new field of endeavour opened up before me; and, after another two years, I am more determined than ever to look for new challenges and to discover areas of life with which I can engage effectively'.

Lastly Ben added something very personal: 'I see a little less (the bleeding affected the optic nerve), but perhaps I hear more acutely – noticeably the birds. And much more that is striking and beautiful, now moves me more. A greater intensity? That sounds good! But when it comes to human suffering and the spoiling of the natural world I sometimes experience a closing down of emotions (as he had put it elsewhere) a loss of moral urgency'.

For me, the two saving factors, providing both mental and physical exercise, were and are the fact that I am a writer and a gardener. After all this time my typing on my loyal Mac, is very inaccurate and still reduced to two fingers, but what is spell check for? I still manage to write a book a year and still (just) manage to grow most of my own fruit and vegetables. In the intervening years I managed, with the help of wheelchairs in airports, to continue travelling both for work and pleasure. What I found was, that if called for, it was possible to do things that I would not have deemed possible, such as being rushed off, on arrival for a conference, on a sightseeing tour of part of Buenos Aires (on foot) by people who would not take no for an answer. Somehow I managed, and enjoyed it, just as one day, in Australia, my grandchildren decided they wanted to explore a deserted beach at the foot of a cliff. Getting down was not too bad, with a helping hand, but getting back up was another matter. We solved it by my daughter placing her foot behind mine at each step to stop me sliding backwards. It was quite a strain but the next day my leg felt stronger than it had been for ages – the effects I suppose of extreme exercise, but I am not sure I would try that particular effort again!

Aids and therapies

There are many things made to help the disabled and most people will have been advised by their therapists on leaving hospital. If a patient is living alone then everything must be done to ensure their safety. Maybe I am just stubborn, but I was sure I would recover eventually and did not want to either be reminded all the time that I was disabled, nor make elaborate changes to our house. Over the years I have discovered others like me as well as those who, not only because of stroke, have quite different views: they have a stairlift put in before they need one, in case, and invest in wet rooms, discarding their old bathrooms.

Over the years I have been very contented with a removeable bath seat and a hand held shower. That left the bath still usable, specially for children in particular. Then a stair lift. I admit it would be helpful for taking loads up and down stairs, but climbing the stairs was the one thing I could manage from the beginning. More importantly, it has been the best strengthening exercise for my leg muscles. However, I eventually succumbed to pressure from kind friends and asked for a visit and estimate, and, as it turns out the space or lack of it at the top and bottom of the stairs makes our house unsuitable for one. Luckily I had not set my heart on it!

I watch my elderly friends enjoying their buggies, and, having tried one while in Australia, know that I would enjoy having one. However, we live out of the town and the kerbs would make life pretty difficult. Also we have nowhere convenient to store it, so while my husband still drives I will forget about it. But there is something more. I recently bought myself something called a rollator – a wonderful object that trundles along with four wheels. It is adjustable and with brakes etc and a basket with cover that acts as a seat. It is just perfect for going up my long garden path, with my bucket and tools on the seat. I immediately felt it saved a lot of tiredness. However, almost immediately, I found myself unable to contemplate going without it. This sudden dependency interests me. Did I wait until the last minute until I could no longer do without it, or have I stopped an effort and exercise that I had always considered beneficial?

This pressure from friends to try this or that therapy has again sometimes been difficult to resist. What well meaning people fail to understand (apart from the cost) is that there might be a benefit but also a price to pay in tiredness and hassle in many of their ideas. There is one important issue that I wrote about in the early part of this book, however, that must be corrected. That concerns acupuncture. Although it did not benefit me early on in my recovery, it was instrumental later on in stabilising the spasms in my legs, and I am extremely grateful to my therapist who persevered. It therefore annoyed me to see a research report that had 'proved' that there was no benefit to stroke patients from acupuncture. As that was dealing only with patients at the very early stage of recovery, I question the methodology. Since then I have heard of other patients who have benefited and hope that no one was put off by what I said ten years ago.

Finally to something I know less about, but one of the saddest consequences of stroke – aphasia. Following on to Ben de la Mare's statement about how people fail to recognise the consequences of stroke, a letter in Stroke News, summer 2011 emphasised this. A stroke survivor wrote of his experience at an airport check-in where he was suspected of drinking because of his slurred speech. It might have resulted in his being refused to fly had he not had a card that he always carried explaining his condition. The Stroke Association now supplies a similar printed card. Anyhow, I had read a certain amount on the subject and visited several groups for the speech impaired, but never really felt there was much I could do to help until a young colleague, a designer, told me that her father, in Argentina, had had a stroke and was suffering from aphasia. His inability to communicate was causing distress to him and his caring family. I had an idea that we could work on together. While speech therapists make use of comprehensive iconic sheets to assist in communication, perhaps something similar and more personal could be devised for use with family or carers in the home. The concept of iconic communication need not be complex. Any mark can be given meaning between any two people. In this case we developed sheets that dealt with the specific tastes and needs of this patient – what he felt like eating or drinking, his favourite music, or what he felt like doing. I was interested in providing what I termed emoticons – something to express what he was feeling like – tired, frustrated, lonely, grateful, etc. His daughter illustrated all these most beautifully, but it would not be necessary to be artistic to do something similar in any home. A simple indicator board, such as suggested to that nurse in Singapore so many years ago (see page 19) would be a start.

We presented this as a joint paper at a conference on Designing Effective Communications in Canada, later to be published. I dealt with the theory and she with the practical aspects. We noticed quite a few people in the audience were reduced to tears, having never envisaged such a condition as severe aphasia.

Just as we all say, it is so much a matter of will power whether or not you can achieve a meaningful life after stroke, nothing helps in your recovery like finding yourself useful again.

References

de la Mare B 2005 *The Experience of Stroke and the Life of the Spirit.* Medical Humanities Vol 31 no 2.

Noel G *Creating Possibilities for Communication.* Designing Effective Communications, ed. J Frascara, Allworth Press.

Sassoon R 2006 *Extending the Boundaries of Communication: Interactive Iconic Communication to Help Those Who Suffer From Aphasia.* Designing Effective Communications, ed. J Frascara, Allworth Press.

Part 2

DIFFERENT PERSPECTIVES

6
The part played
by the contributors

MOST OF THOSE who have contributed to the second part of this book are part of my own story of recovery and discovery. The account starts with my attempts to find a walking aid to replace the ill-fitting splint that came out of a cupboard in hospital, and was only meant as a temporary safety measure. I felt it was impeding rather than aiding my progress. Enquiries led me to the orthotist at the district hospital the day my original physiotherapist (see page 26) was asking for volunteers to take part in a training day to be run by the team from Salisbury on the use of the Odstock Dropped Foot Stimulator (ODFS). One thing led to another and a couple of months later I was accepted on the programme described by Paul Taylor and Jane Burridge on page 81.

To be part of a research project is, in itself, an enormous boost to any patient's morale. To meet people whose expertise is so evident gives you hope, apart from the obvious practical consequences. The first trial with the ODFS at Salisbury Hospital showed a dramatic improvement in my walking speed. However, I had the feeling that it would not be good for me if the device took over the act of lifting my dropped foot all the time. (It was only at Salisbury that the term 'drop-foot' was finally explained to me.) It was agreed that I should use the device only half of the time, even though at that time there was no evidence that there was a carry-over effect (i.e. that it would help my muscles to learn to do the job themselves). I always felt, however, that an echo remained to activate those muscles for an instant, after the switch was turned off. It is difficult to separate the effects of the odfs in retraining my leg to help itself, and the other factors involved. Using the device reminded me of how it felt to walk naturally again and helped to lengthen my stride from the typical short, tentative steps of the stroke patient. Then a growing confidence in my ability to move without tripping over at each step encouraged more walking. All this contributed, over a period of about a year, to the gradual strengthening of my whole leg until it seemed time to make it do its own work. I am convinced that the Odstock Dropped Foot Stimulator contributed considerably to the speed of my recovery, although I cannot claim to have contributed much to research in return. However, it was interesting to learn that now the opinion is that patients should not use the device full time, to avoid the problem of becoming overdependent on it.

A gait analysis

The next episode took place in Australia. For many years we have spent part of the (northern) winter in Perth and I have had friendly contact with the department of Human Movement in the University of Western Australia. Some nine months after my stroke we took the risk of keeping to our usual habit, only to find that flying half way around the world was considerably easier than taking a commuter train from our local station to London. You are given a wheel-chair (which is still necessary because of the distance in airports) and looked after at every stage of the journey.

I took my equipment to the department to show it off, and was rewarded by an offer to do a comparative gait analysis with and without the fes (Functional Electrical Stimulation). This test consists of fixing markers on strategic points of my body and limbs so that they appear on the computer, allowing a complete picture of my movements. Speed, force and cadence were among the factors measured. Although I did not appreciate it at the time, reading it again now I can see how many details it revealed – the weakness of my knee and upper leg that I eventually realised myself, and used an inexpensive pedal machine to strengthen, and the need to lengthen my stride that still needs more work today – and much more.

Incidentally, on the same day as the gait analysis another vital service was offered. Curtin University runs a driving assessment centre fully equipped with simulators and other testing equipment. At that time I was worried that, in order to keep my licence from being taken away, there was a test to be taken on returning home. This centre provided an opportunity to find out how I was likely to perform, away from the tension of an actual test situation. It pinpointed what aspects needed to improve and was a great relief. Such centres are also available throughout Great Britain.

Practical therapy at last

Pete Hamer and David Lloyd's detailed gait analysis awaited me on our return to England, but it was more than six months later before Jane Cast (see page 73) could interpret it properly for me. She is an experienced community neurophysiotherapist and was fully occupied at that time working locally for Cheshire Homes. Like my Australian friends, she was shocked by the condition that I had been left in. She could not offer me intensive therapy and rather doubted whether I would, by myself, be able to correct the bent posture and awkward gait that I had adopted. She gave a detailed explanation of my condition and the precise purpose of each of the exercises she prescribed. This, combined with my own shock at realising how bad I had let my whole situation become, made me discipline myself to keep to a fairly rigid regime. For the first time I found how satisfying systematic exercise was, and how quickly results could be seen. It took only three informal visits over a period of perhaps six weeks to get me upright, and transferring my weight properly from one foot to another.

There are several conclusions to draw from this from the patient's angle:

1. Therapists cannot take it for granted that a positive reply means that a patient understands all that they are being told, for example that they understand terms such as tone, or that the patients, when optimists, are really as far recovered as they appear.

2. How easy it is and how dangerous to get the balance wrong between regaining function and learning good movement.

3. How difficult it is for people to realise when they are not upright with their weight evenly balanced, or to work out quite obvious strategies that would benefit them.

4. How difficult it is to self-correct without guidance, but how quickly results can come from just a little clear expert advice.

5. How, with expert help, it is never too late to retrain and improve.

Perhaps we have both helped each other, because the speed with which her exercise regime changed my life has encouraged her to take on more long-term, neglected patients. Jane had found the same kind of results which she reports in her section starting on page 73. I learned that it is the precise description of how an exercise should be carried out, and what its purpose is, allied to the placing of the body correctly so that you can feel what is correct, that allows you to help yourself. The attitude of the therapist makes a huge difference. He or she needs to show a difficult mix of positive encouragement and firmness. Above all the patient needs to feel that therapists know what they are doing and that they really care about achieving a result. There must be a mutual respect, with the patient's views and wishes taken into account. Exercises insufficiently explained and given too early, before people have the strength to do them properly, may cause them to lose faith in exercise altogether. The episode of the gait analysis emphasised how difficult it is to self-correct, and how essential an expert intervention is, irrespective of the stage of recovery.

Jane was just starting her new job as Stroke Care Co-ordinator, across South West Kent Primary Care Trust. This includes collecting relevant data, surveying existing local services to see how they can be improved and looking at examples of good practice in other trusts. These activities should be taking place in health authorities country-wide in conjunction with the National Service Framework (NFS) for Older People (see page 129) and the clinical guidelines of the Royal College of Physicians.

Occupational therapy

I had little personal experience of good practice in occupational therapy during my recovery, although the safety equipment recommended and demonstrated by the OT department helped me considerably on my return home. The shower seat was particularly successful and I still use it. The therapy that was provided might have been sufficient for the very elderly who needed only the most basic skills in the home, but lacked understanding of anyone needing any more. I am not being critical of the teaching of essential daily living skills and realise that they are very important, particularly for patients who will be living alone. I am making a plea for a bit more thought about individual needs. Having once, at an earlier stage of my professional life, fought for signature writing to be included as a daily living skill, it seems to me that there now needs to be further advances in that area, to equip patients for a fuller and more satisfying life once they are back in their own homes.

My first priority, admittedly rather unusual, was assurance that I would be able to manipulate a keyboard one-handed.

A request to try that instead of tea making was met with incredulity. Yet computers play such a vital part in most people's lives, surely it is time to consider them more seriously. Apart from the fact that many disabled people may become dependent on computers to communicate, even to do their daily shopping, the use of a keyboard is excellent therapy (with instant feedback in terms of increasing accuracy, just like handwriting). It may be difficult for older therapists to appreciate how widely and naturally their patients will have used computers. They (the therapists) may feel threatened by something they do not wholly understand. Patients may also need guidance about more specialised technology to help them in their new life (or at least information as to where to access this).

I am aware that there is an acute shortage of occupational therapists in our part of the world and that, in all fairness, with constant staff changes the whole ethos of a department can alter considerably over a period of time.

Speech and language therapy

I did not have, or witness, any speech and language therapy, although the need for a speech therapist in the rehabilitation unit was obvious. It was by chance that I met Deborah Harding (see page 93), when our train to London was delayed one morning, and we soon discovered our mutual interest. A Registered Member of the Royal College of Speech and Language Therapists she has practised as a speech and language therapist in the field of adult neurorehabilitation, having first completed an M.Sc. in Cognitive Neuropsychology at the University of London. She has published papers in the area of cognitive neuro-psychological approaches to aphasia therapy, as well as writing on broader service delivery issues. She currently manages a multi-disciplinary team at West Kent Neurorehabilitation Unit. A member of the British Aphasiology Society, she served for six years as Secretary to the Society.

Bobath technique

The link with the article by Dr Mayston (see page 88) on the Bobath technique dates back to my early days in hospital. One of the young physiotherapists had returned from an advanced Bobath course. The techniques she had learned were an immediate advance, felt by patients and the others who gathered round to learn. How I agree with these sentences from the Bobath concept (see page 89), on the part motivation also plays when being set and achieving meaningful and relevant goals:

> 'While it was thought that teaching people normal move-ment patterns and postural reactions would automatically lead to the performance of functional tasks, it is now known that the activity of the cns is task dependent (Flament et al, 1993 and Ehrsson, et al 2000). Therefore it is essential that therapists work with clients to achieve goals that are relevant to their lives, and not goals decided for them by therapists.'

Doctors' attitudes

Professor McLellan, who was Great Britain's first professor of rehabilitation, needs no introduction to anyone in the field. I was fortunate to visit his department in Southampton several years before my stroke. His sensitive contribution describes the changing attitudes of doctors as they are trained in rehabilitation medicine. One matter he stresses is that: 'While two strokes may appear much the same, two people with strokes never are, and that the attributes and objectives of the person who has a stroke are crucial elements in negotiating what rehabilitation should aim at, and what form it should take.'

The ARNI approach to functional recovery from stroke

I met Tom Balchin after the publication of the first edition of this book, and partly as a result of it, because of both of our

71

involvement in stroke rehabilitation. He describes the concepts and techniques of the organisation that he founded, Action for the Rehabilitation from Neurological Injury, in order to help stroke survivors in a structured way, including the theory of neural plasticity.

Ten years on we have tried to contact all the original contributors. A couple we could not trace, and some were happy to leave their parts unchanged. Others have brought their contributions up to date. Professor Alan Wing and his colleagues have kindly contributed an entirely new chapter.

It seems that those who have contributed to this part of the book share many similar views.

7

Physiotherapy: the importance of a physical management plan

JANE CAST

A S A PHYSIOTHERAPIST with an interest in neurology, particularly the issues arising from those with a long term disability, the importance of an ongoing management plan in their daily lives has become apparent to me. It is devastating to see someone who has suffered from a stroke, told the diagnosis, admitted to hospital for varying amounts of rehabilitation, then literally cast into the community and left to get on with it. There is so much ongoing rehabilitation that could help people to reach their full potential, yet it seems there is a cut-off point when everyone assumes that there is nothing more that can be done. People are left wondering why no one shows any more interest. They feel entirely on their own with no further guidance as to what they might achieve.

Treating neurological patients in the community has revealed how little rehabilitation can be offered to those in certain areas of the country. People who wish to try and improve their physical capabilities generally have no plan of action once they get back home. Out-patient or community physiotherapy may be arranged for a short time only. If not, it may be assumed that they will continue to improve without further assistance and direction. This also means that some will deteriorate with no further input and possibly return back to the hospital. An unnecessary pattern of crisis management may then develop. This reminds me of a patient who had a mild stroke and was not judged to need any physiotherapy on discharge from hospital. When she was seen a few years later after several falls and failing to cope at home the results of this neglect were apparent. One-sided, with significant balance problems and the inability to transfer weight successfully, she needed much more intensive treatment to overcome these acquired disabilities.

People often do not realise how their condition has changed. When questioned about what exercises they are doing they may reply: 'The ones shown in hospital' – even if this was several years after! Aids given out initially may now no longer be needed. Patients have no guidelines to follow and fear a deterioration if they change anything. It could be that the complete opposite is true for some. The body may be allowed to recruit more normal movement patterns when an aid is withdrawn. With ongoing recovery people deserve more under-standing of how to manage their condition. They need to understand how modifying their efforts and using normal patterns of movement will help to promote further recovery.

Everyone should realise that patients can continue to improve long after their stroke. I recently visited a patient some two years after his stroke. Without ongoing treatment he was confined to a wheelchair. The complicating factor was his height; he was six foot four. He had mastered transfers but nobody had had the courage to try to get him to walk. We made it a challenge and worked out a friendly 'contract', allowing him, initially, to set the timescale. Intermediate goals were the next stage, proving the patient's own estimate to have been highly pessimistic. He is still making good progress towards walking.

Physiotherapy does not need to be daily, weekly or even monthly, however, there should be somebody involved who has a particular interest in neurology. These are the people best able to assess and re-assess each individual's needs. They can give patients new goals, set new programmes, explore new challenges as well as offer patients the motivation and support they need to believe they can become more functionally independent. This, for most people, is their aim, but a lack of specialised physiotherapists can make accessing their service difficult.

Ongoing help

A stroke comes as a devastating event and initially people are unable to fully appreciate the extent of the damage. That realisation will not come until a much later stage. It is important that at this point they receive informed, positive help to look to the future. An encouraging attitude can help to alleviate depression and combat the fear that this is how they are destined to live the rest of their lives. People need informed help to enable them to focus on what they are trying to achieve and to analyse how best to approach the task. This can be neglected in hospital, as time constraints are very difficult.

Stroke management at home, once they are medically stable and able to transfer, can offer advantages. They are in a familiar environment so it is easier to identify more realistic goals. Patients start to understand how they can take more responsibility for their own recovery. Working at home allows simple exercises to be incorporated into daily activities. In this way the constant reinforcement of exercises and positioning throughout the day has a long lasting beneficial effect – as long as they are done correctly. The patient can be given an uninterrupted one-to-one session, which is often not possible in a busy out-patient department or ward. Patients may also feel more at ease to express their worries and identify more specific activities that are a problem in their home environment. These can then be assessed and a plan of action implemented to either improve or alter their activity.

The physiotherapist plays an important role in educating people about the potential they have and then encouraging them to reach out to achieve goals that otherwise they might have thought impossible. Positive feedback can only help to further their drive and desire to make more effort themselves. The more they achieve the more likely they are to want to do more. Lack of input or a challenge can lead to deterioration, low morale and poor outcome. It is amazing how a few simple words of advice can help to move somebody on to the next stage.

Another function of a physiotherapist is multidisciplinary working and liaison to ensure that all the patient's needs are adequately met. The importance of the role of the carer should also be considered; he or she can make a huge difference. An enthusiastic new carer gave Mary a new lease of life fifteen years after her stroke. Spending time with her, showing her a few simple positions, how to stretch and involve her hand in daily exercises allowed Mary to move her fingers at long last. For therapists and carers alike it is extremely satisfying to work with those in the community whose needs have been neglected, and to give them new hope. A team approach should enable patients to achieve independence in many aspects of life.

The benefits of talking to professionals cannot be under-estimated. They have the vital experience and knowledge of appropriate treatments, aids and adaptations. An ongoing physical management plan can be developed following discussion and assessment, looking at a broad spectrum of activities. This should be reviewed at regular intervals and adjusted as necessary. Any plan needs to take into account what is available in the locality but should be tailored to suit each individual's need. The emphasis should be on appropriate advice, education and treatment. Some form of supervision will be required to ensure that the plan is being followed correctly and its goals fulfilled.

Areas that are often neglected

Through working with a broad spectrum of neurological patients it is possible to observe certain common areas of neglect that frequently occur. This can lead to reduced functional ability, unnecessary pain and weakness in joints and muscles, which in turn prevent patients from developing their full physical potential.

The concept of normal movement sequences, tone and balance are key factors around which stroke recovery and rehabilitation are based. It is therefore vital that the patients are given time for a detailed explanation of what they are trying to achieve while the therapists are working with them to facilitate the movement. If patients and carers appreciate what they are aiming at, or at least what they are expected to do, they are far more likely to succeed. This can also prevent the development of a series of secondary complications, through misunderstanding the complex physical effects of the stroke.

The emphasis on rehabilitation can often be on getting the patient to transfer and walk in order to be able to return home. This may result in a neglected arm and hand. In the meantime patients can become increasingly skilled at managing all activities one handed and so the full potential of the affected one is never developed.

The arm can be a source of many problems. Patients frequently experience loss of movement – and therefore loss of function – as well as varying degrees of pain. It can be a long and gradual process awaiting any return of active movement in the arm. Meanwhile, much can be done to encourage patients to adopt an appropriate management plan. This should ensure that they do not lose vital ranges of movement, and also should promote a bilateral approach.

The positioning of the arm, both in bed and sitting in the chair, is important. This is in order to normalise tone or to protect an arm with low tone. It is also relevant when there is loss of sensation and neglect. Joints should be kept as mobile as possible and handled very carefully. Pain, contractures, subluxation of the shoulder, loss of range of movement, or stiffness, can all develop quite quickly. Everything possible needs to be done to prevent these problems. Associated reactions in the upper limb should also be addressed because these will have an effect on other activities such as gait.

Pain is often prevalent in the upper limb and may be reduced by proper management in the early stages particularly. This includes correct positioning, teaching specific exercises, encouraging the person to look after the arm, as well as passive mobilisations and stretches. There are various other techniques which may be used in the management of the upper limb, such as functional electrical stimulation, splints and positioning aids. Botulinum toxin can be helpful in some cases to control spasticity.

The trunk (the bit in the middle!) is sometimes forgotten, but is of vital importance as it provides a stable base for both the upper, lower limbs and head to work from. People are frequently left sitting in inappropriate chairs without correct support, thereby reinforcing abnormal patterns of movement and allowing the trunk to become weak and ineffective. A wheelchair can be a useful piece of equipment in the short/long term because it can provide a good sitting posture and may allow more freedom of movement.

The trunk may also have difficulty functioning correctly if the patient has been given a walking aid too early. By allowing someone to fix on to a stick or tripod, the whole dynamics of walking can alter. It is often very difficult to withdraw the aid at a late date when that person may feel unable to manage without it. High sticks can be useful for providing stability without compromising on posture. Simple activities such as rolling and unsupported sitting, may enable the trunk to become more mobile.

Lower limbs also require careful management and positioning in a similar way to the arm. It is particularly important to prevent tightness developing around the hip, knee and ankle. These can all affect the gait pattern quite markedly. Appropriate footwear is needed to provide correct support and stability. Some people may need more specialist advice with this, perhaps intervention from an orthotist, to help them to gain a stable base for weight bearing.

Bad habits or new problems can develop at any time. It is the role of neurological physiotherapists to analyse these changes.

They can then help to develop a plan. This would integrate such treatment as is available locally with careful guidance to the patient. This would be aimed at highlighting their role in their own recovery. A more positive outcome will always occur where there is appropriate support and explanation to stroke patients from those who are involved in their care.

Ten years on and I continue to thoroughly enjoy the challenge and fulfilment gained from treating patients with neurological problems. I am currently working at the West Kent Neuro Rehab Unit which specialises in treating people with acquired brain injury.

My passionate belief that there is always scope for improvement remains central to my ethos of treatment and patient's deteriorations can often be just caused by their lack of confidence or low self esteem. I still use management plans, finding them a very simple but incredibly powerful tool to motivate and improve patients. I have now developed a template which once completed for the individual allows them to comprehend very specifically their own personal difficulties and then details methods to address these. Other areas that have informed/developed my practice come from a variety of settings. From my present job I have learnt the benefits of demanding that patients work hard and perform to a high standard, thereby achieving their goals. The recent implementation of constraint induced therapy to help regain function of the weaker arm has shown some great results with just two weeks intensive practice. The therapists also assess carefully the possible need for appropriate supports or orthotics. These can make a significant change to the quality of functional movement and the management of joint positioning and pain.

I have taken up Iyengar yoga, learning in great detail about alignment of the body and the need for good posture flexibility and strength. Transferring these skills into treatment sessions with stroke patients has proved to be very beneficial.

My focus on solving the problem of a lack of independence in patients, coupled with their inability to access the community, has led me to take a much more proactive approach. I positively encourage patients wherever relevant to use aids, electric wheelchairs, adapted cars etc if it gives them the independence that so many of them wish for.

My last thought and this has to be one for all stroke patients to work towards. Believe strongly in your ability to achieve and set your long term sights high. I have just returned from the Base Camp of Everest with a patient and yes it wasn't easy but we did it and so can you.

8

Functional Electrical Stimulation – the Odstock Dropped Foot Stimulator

PAUL TAYLOR AND JANE BURRIDGE

Functional electrical stimulation (FES) was first used by the American bioengineer, W T Liberson, to help people who had had a stroke to lift their affected foot when walking. For some time after this the idea was not developed mainly because the technology was neither reliable nor user-friendly. The principle of FES is to replace the nerve impulses that are interrupted by damage to the brain or spinal cord with small electrical signals. It can be used not only with people who have had a stroke, but also people with spinal cord or head injuries, MS or cerebral palsy. It seems that it is particularly useful when people have spasticity – muscle stiffness.

Since Liberson's time there has been a considerable global research effort, the majority of which has been aimed at systems to help the spinal cord injured. However, more recently, attention has been turned towards stroke and some systems are beginning to become available. During the last fifteen years research at the Salisbury District Hospital has been attempting to make fes more effective and useful, by developing equipment and the clinical techniques and service. The people who are most likely to benefit are those who have a drop-foot, that causes them either to trip or hitch their hip when they walk. Work is also being done to apply the techniques to be useful with people who have some arm function but who, for example, lack the ability to open the hand even though they have quite a good grip.

Drop-foot

Drop-foot following stroke is a common problem. The condition prevents the patient from effectively swinging the leg when walking, causing an abnormal gait. The increased effort required not only means that walking is slow, tiring and sometimes unsafe, due to tripping, but may lead to further increase in spasticity.

Drop-foot is conventionally corrected by splinting, usually by a plastic ankle foot orthosis and, occasionally, a more substantial splint attached to the shoe. Many patients find the splint uncomfortable, sometimes exacerbating ankle oedema. In some cases patients do not find splinting an effective way of overcoming drop-foot, it may in fact lead to a further increase in calf tone and other problems.

The Odstock Dropped Foot Stimulator (ODFS) is a single-channel, foot-switch-triggered stimulator designed to elicit dorsiflexion of the foot by stimulation of the common peroneal nerve and is a direct development of a device first described by Liberson. The stimulator is about the size of a pack of cards and can be worn at the waist on a belt, or in a pocket. Leads connect the stimulator to the switch and the electrodes on the leg. Self-adhesive skin-surface electrodes are placed over the common peroneal nerve as it passes over the head of the fibula bone and the motor point, that is where the nerve enters the muscle, of tibialis anterior. The rise and fall of the stimulation can be adjusted to prevent a stretch reflex in the calf muscles, which is a significant component of spasticity. The device after a few days of practice, can be used all day as an orthotic aid or a training aid in gait re-education.

The ODFS was the subject of a randomised controlled trial (rct) in which 32 stroke patients who had had a stroke for in excess of six months were allocated to a treatment group or a control group. The treatment group used the device and also received 12 sessions of physiotherapy, while the control group, who received the same contact time, only received physiotherapy. After three months of use the treatment group showed a statistically significant increase in walking speed and a reduction in the physiological cost index (pci) when the stimulator was used, while no changes were seen in the control group. No significant 'carry-over' effect was seen, although a trend was present. Users of the odfs showed a continuing reduction in quadriceps spasticity, which was only seen in the control group while physiotherapy continued. The treatment group also showed a reduction in the Hospital Anxiety and Depression index, suggesting an improvement in quality of life which was not seen in the control group. Of the 32 subjects at the start of the trial, eight were using a splint, 13 had rejected this means of correction and 11 had either been advised not to use it or had not been offered it. All subjects in this trial who used electrical stimulation to correct drop-foot continued with this method in preference to conventional splinting.

The trial results were presented to the South and West Development and Evaluation Committee who, after examining this and evidence from other groups, subsequently recommended the odfs for use in the UK's National Health Service.

Following the establishment of a clinical service, it was decided to continue recording the main outcome measures of walking speed and pci that had been recorded in the rct. An audit of these parameters over the first 18 weeks of use, confirmed the results of the original rct and also showed a significant carry-over effect, i.e. an improvement in walking ability when not using the stimulator, in a group of 111 stroke subjects. A questionnaire survey indicated that the most common reasons for using the device were that it reduced the effort of walking, reduced tripping and improved confidence. Compliance was 92 per cent at 18 weeks and 86 per cent at one year. In the year 2000 the device was recommended by the Royal College of Physicians in their publication *National clinical guidelines on stroke*.

Other uses of the stimulators

While the odfs is effective for many users, there often remains other gait problems. These can be addressed by stimulating additional muscle groups. A second device, the Odstock 2 Channel Stimulator, has been developed for this purpose. By stimulation of the hamstrings, knee flexion can be improved or the gluteus maximus muscle can be used to give hip extension while weight bearing. Other applications include bilateral dropped-foot and the stimulation of the triceps muscle to improve arm swing and, therefore, balance in gait. Another development, which is in the preliminary trial stages, is an implanted dropped-foot stimulator. Two different approaches are currently being investigated. The first, from Holland, uses a two channel implanted stimulator, one channel for each branch of the common peroneal nerve. In this way it is possible to independently control the amount of dorsiflexion (foot lift) and eversion (foot twisting outwards) allowing an accurate control of the foot's movements. Like the ODFS this device uses a foot switch. A second approach, this time from Denmark, uses a multi-channel nerve cuff on the common peroneal nerve, which again allows selection of different movements. A novel feature of this system is that the researchers plan to pick up nerve signals from the sole of the foot to detect when the foot is placed on, or taken off, the floor. This has been shown to work in the laboratory but as yet is not available for home use.

Further research

Research is also being done to attempt to improve hand, arm and shoulder function. Shoulder subluxation is a common problem following stroke and is due to the inability of the shoulder muscles to maintain the humerus bone in its socket. This is often associated with pain. It has been shown that exercising using electrical stimulation, can reduce the subluxation and often eliminate shoulder pain. Similar exercises are also used for the hand and it has been shown that the voluntary range of movement can be improved and spasticity can be reduced. Anecdotally it has been claimed that these exercises can improve hand function, hastening recovery and it has also been suggested that sensory ability may also be improved.

Research is under way in several centres to produce a functional orthosis for the hand that would work in a similar way to the odfs. At the time of writing, these devices have not entered regular clinical service, but promise useful benefit in the future. One approach is to use sensitive amplifiers to pick the residual electrical activity from the partially paralysed muscles and use this to control electrical stimulation, boosting the activity of the muscle. Other systems have suggested using other body-worn sensors to detect the user's intention to open their hand. As with drop-foot, implanted systems are also being considered.

Since the original article was written the use of FES for correction of dropped foot has become more established in clinical practice. There are now two additional devices on the UK market, the Bioness L300 and the WalkAide system and the ODFS III device has been updated becoming the ODFS Pace. In 2009 the National Institute for Health and Clinical Excellence published guidelines for the use of FES to correct dropped foot using both implanted and external systems and recommended its use for the NHS. In 2010 the NHS Purchasing and Supplies Agency produced a series of reports on Functional Electrical Stimulation for Dropped Foot of Central Neurological Origin. The *Economic Review* describes a cost benefit model for the technique and demonstrates that the ODFS was cost effective for the NHS.

Our work to improve hand and arm function following stroke has continued. In 2011 we published the results of a pilot trial that examined the use of a FES device for opening the hand and extending the elbow, triggered by a movement sensor. Significant improvements in function were reported after three months treatment and these were maintained three months after the treatment was withdrawn. A larger scale randomized controlled trial (REAcH) is currently underway to verify the results, funded by the Stroke Association.

For more information about FES clinical service and research in Salisbury District Hospital with many links to other FES sites please check our web site: www.salisburyfes.com

References

1   Liberson W, Holmquest H, Scott M. 'Functional electrotherapy: stimulation of the common peroneal nerve synchronised with the swing phase of gait of hemiplegic subjects', *Archives of Physical Medicine and Rehabilitation*, 1961, 42, pp. 202–5.

2   Burridge J, Taylor P, Hagan S, Swain I. 'Experience of clinical use of the Odstock Dropped Foot Stimulator', *Artificial Organs*, 1997, 21(3), pp. 254–60.

3   Burridge J, Taylor P, Hagan S, Wood D, Swain I. 'The effects of common peroneal nerve stimulation on the effort and speed of walking: a randomised controlled clinical trial with chronic hemiplegic patients', *Clinical Rehabilitation*, 1997, 11, pp. 201–10.

4   Burridge J, Taylor P, Hagan S A, Wood D E, Swain I D. 'The effect on the spasticity of the quadriceps muscles of stimulation of the common peroneal nerve of chronic hemiplegic subjects during walking'. *Physiotherapy*, 1997, vol. 83, no 2.

5   Taylor P N, Burridge J H, Wood D E, Norton J, Dunkerly A, Singleton, C, Swain I D. 'Clinical use of the Odstock Drop Foot Stimulator – its effect on the speed and effort of walking', *Archives of Physical Medicine and Rehabilitation*, 1999, 80, pp. 1577–83.

6   Benson K and Hartz A J. 'A comparison of observational studies and randomized controlled trials', *N Engl J Med*, 2000, 342, pp. 1878–86.

7   Taylor P N, Burridge J H, Dunkerley A L, Lamb A, Wood D E, Norton J A, Swain I D. 'Patient's Perceptions of the Odstock Dropped Foot Stimulator (ODFS)', *Clinical Rehabilitation*, 1999, 13, pp. 333–40.

8   Intercollegiate working party for stroke. 'National clinical guidelines for stroke', 2000, London, Royal College of Physicians, (ISBN 1860 161 200).

9   Baker L L, Yeh C, Wilson D, Waters R L. 'Electrical stimulation of wrist and fingers for hemiplegic patients', Physical Therapy, 1979, 59 (12), pp. 1495–9.

10   Pandyan A D, Granat M H. 'Effects of electrical stimulation on flexion contractures in hemiplegics', Clinical Rehabilitation, 1997, 11, pp. 123–30.

11   Bowman B R, Baker L L, Waters R L. 'Position feedback and electrical stimulation: an automated treatment for hemiplegic wrist', Archives of Physical Medicines and Rehabilitation, Nov. 1979, Vol. 60, pp. 497–501.

12   Kraft G H, Fitts S S and Hammond, M C. 'Techniques to improve function of the arm and hand in chronic hemiplegia', Archives of Physical Medicines and Rehabilitation, 1992, 73, pp. 220–7.

13   Prada G, Tallis R. 'Treatment of the neglect syndrome in stroke patients using a contingency stimulator', Clinical Rehabilitation, 1995, 9, pp. 304–13.

14   Functional electrical stimulation for drop foot of central neurological origin N1733 1P ISBN 84629-846-6, Jan 09. http://www.nice.org.uk/Guidance/IPG278

15   Treating drop foot using electrical stimulation N1734 1P ISBN 1-84629-847-4, Jan 09. http://www.nice.org.uk/Guidance/IPG278

16   Economic Report. Functional Electrical Stimulation for dropped foot of central neurological origin. CEP10012 Published by the NHS Purchasing and Supply Agency, Feb 2010 www.dh.gov.uk/cep

17   Mann G, Taylor P, Lane R. Accelerometer-triggered electrical stimulation for reach and grasp in chronic stroke patients: a pilot study. Neurorehabil Neural Repair. 2011, Oct; 25(8):774-80. Epub 31 May 2011.

9
The Bobath Concept*

MARGARET J MAYSTON

FOLLOWING THE RETIREMENT of Mrs Bobath from clinical practice and teaching in the late 1980s, there has been little or no literature by Bobath tutors to explain changes in philosophy or practice. The most commonly quoted reference to support Bobath as applied to the management of adults is the third and last edition of *Adult Hemiplegia* (Bobath, 1990). Similarly, for paediatrics the usually quoted work is Bobath and Bobath (1975).

According to these, the Bobath Concept uses the analysis of movement to determine what is necessary and possible for a client to achieve. The treatment ideas employed by the Bobaths were based on the knowledge available at the time, and assumed that spasticity was a problem of overactivity of the muscles resulting from abnormally enhanced tonic reflex activity. Accordingly it was thought that handling techniques inhibited such activity and made it possible for the person to achieve more normal movement.

Since then our understanding of the control of movement and spasticity has progressed. We know that tone, whether it is normal or abnormal, comprises both neural and non-neural components. Spasticity, classically referred to by Lance (1980) as a velocity-dependent increase in tonic stretch reflexes, is only

*This section is based on 'Motor Learning Now Needs Meangingful Goals'. *Physiotherapy* September 2000/vol 86/no 9

one component of the movement dysfunction that may be encountered by people with neurological impairment, and in fact probably contributes very little to their movement disabilities.

Handling by itself cannot change spasticity (which represents the neural component of hypertonia), but may result in improved muscle length to allow for more efficient muscle activation. It is only by enabling the person to move more actively in more optimal and meaningful ways within the limits of their Central Nervous System damage that any reduction in the negative effects of spasticity can be achieved. While handling can be important in effecting changes in visco-elastic properties of muscle, activity is the key. It is not possible to effect normal activity in a cns which has been significantly damaged, but the therapist can work with the client to optimise the remaining cns tissue. The advances in neural plasticity, in particular the work of Nudo et al (see Nudo 1998 for a review) highlight the importance of activity to drive neuroplastic changes within the cns. Therapists cannot directly inhibit spasticity (see Mayston 2002), but they can and must teach their clients to move in more efficient and functional ways.

Mrs Bobath at all times stressed the importance of activity, stating that although the handling was important, unless you make the person active you have 'done nothing at all'. (Bobath 1965). There is no good evidence to show that stopping a person from being active will prevent spasticity. This cannot be justified on scientific or financial grounds.

However, it should not be any activity. While it was thought that teaching people normal movement patterns and postural reactions would automatically lead to the performance of functional tasks, it is now known that the activity of the cns is task dependent (Flament et al, 1993 and Ehrsson et al 2000). Therefore it is essential that therapists work with clients to achieve goals that are relevant to their lives, and not goals decided for them by therapists.

Bobath stressed the importance of common sense and using 'what works'. Changes in both the understanding of the neurologically impaired person and the recognition that clinical presentations are often more complex than those clients on whom Mrs Bobath based her clinical observations and formulated her approach, also necessitates the need to modify clinical practice. The use of splints is not contra-indicated, but is seen as an adjunct to therapy, and can facilitate more efficient activity in other body parts. In addition, the use of pharmacological agents such as botulinum toxin, and other adjuncts such as functional electrical stimulation and muscle strengthening when used as a part of the process of achieving optimal functional ability of the person, can also be of value (Damiano and Abel 1998; Miller and Light, 1997).

Bobath-trained therapists are aware of the three main principles of motor learning:

1. Active participation

2. Opportunities for practice

3. Meaningful goals

The first two have always been important aspects of the application of the Bobath concept, but it is only in recent years that the importance of meaningful goals has been emphasised. Perhaps Bobath therapists have become so enthusiastic about changing tone that they have neglected the need to activate clients in meaningful ways.

Bobath-trained therapists have excellent knowledge of the analysis of movement, a skill which can be complemented by current objective biomechanical and neurophysiological measures of joint range, force output, reflex activity and muscle tone, in addition to the appropriate functional outcome measures. Therapists can then more effectively help clients achieve their optimal potential.

Where does this leave Bobath therapists? Is it time to

recognise that we should acknowledge Mrs Bobath as a pioneer who was instrumental in changing clinical practice by recognising that every neurologically impaired person has a potential for improved activity in the affected body parts? Should we now go forwards, and not call what we do Bobath? Perhaps those who consider that they have taken the Bobath ideas forwards should consider putting their own names (or another name) to what they do and teach. Can we recognise the Bobath Centre as an important place to commemorate the contribution that Dr and Mrs Bobath made to neuro-rehabilitation, but realise that what is done within its walls attempts to encompass current knowledge and give clients their best possible chance to lead a better quality of life?

I speak as Director of the Bobath Centre when I state that we are not inhibiting abnormal reflexes, facilitating postural reactions and preventing clients from moving in ways which we think will increase their abnormal tone. Rather we work for optimal length and activity of muscles in a functional context, working with clients and families to determine what goals will improve the quality of life of all concerned. It is a process which requires ongoing self-education and evaluation.

References

Bobath B. 'Notes on Reflex Inhibiting Postures', archival material, Bobath Centre, London.

Bobath B. *Adult hemiplegia: Education and Treatment*, Heinemann Medical Books, 1990, Oxford, 3rd ed.

Bobath B and Bobath K. *Motor development in Different Types of Cerebral Palsy*, Heinemann Medical Books, Oxford, 1975.

Damiano D L and Abel L F. 'Functional Outcomes of Strength Training in Spastic Cerebral Palsy', *Archives of Physical Medicine and Rehabilitation*, 1998, 79, 2, pp. 119–25.

Ehrsson H H, Fagergren A, Jonsson T, Westling G, Johansson R and Forssberg H. 'Cortical activity in precision versus power grip tasks: an MRI study', *Journal of Neurophysiology*, 2000, 83, 1, pp. 528–36.

Flament D, Goldsmith P, Buckley J C, and Lemon R N. 'Task-dependence of EMG responses in first dorsal interosseous muscle to magnetic brain stimulation in man', *Journal of Physiology*, London, 2000, 464, pp. 361–72.

Lance J W. Symposium Synopsis. In 'Spasticity: Disordered Motor Control'. Editors: Feldman R G, Young R R, and Koella W O. *Chicago Year Book of Medical Publishers*, 1980, pages 485–95.

Mayston M J. 'Setting the scene' in: Edwards S (ed). *Neurological Physiotherapy: A problem solving approach*, Churchill Livingstone, Edinburgh, 2002, 2nd ed.

Miller G J T and Light K E. 'Strength training in spastic hemiparesis: Should it be avoided?', *Neurorehabilitation* 9, 1997, pp. 17–28.

Nudo R. 'Role of cortical plasticity in motor recovery after stroke', *Neurology Report*, 1998, 22, pp. 61–7.

10
When words don't work – what to expect from speech and language therapy

DEBORAH HARDING

JUST TAKE A FEW MINUTES out to imagine yourself on a holiday overseas. It's a place where you do not speak the language very well but you are able to get by with a bit of rusty vocabulary you learnt at school and a phrase book. Unexpectedly you wake up in a hospital bed on a busy ward. You feel pretty groggy. There are tubes and charts all around. A nurse arrives, smiles and begins to talk to you. She speaks so fast. You think you caught a few words you recognised but can't quite remember what they mean. You think of things you want to ask – you've noticed your right arm and leg seem heavy and numb, you've got a headache, but how on earth do you understand what is going on? The few things you do manage to say are met with puzzled looks – your pronunciation's not up to much and after a few attempts your confidence is ebbing away and you're beginning to feel pretty anxious about speaking. It's scary and it's isolating and it resembles a little the experience of aphasia, the loss of language often associated with a left hemisphere stroke. Worse still for the person with aphasia, when family and friends turn up to visit they all seem to be speaking that strange, vaguely recognisable, language and they can't make any sense of what the patient is saying to them. (For fuller personal accounts see ref. 1.) At this point, hopefully, the friendly, smiling nurse reaches for the phone and makes a referral to the speech and language therapy department.

Communication and swallowing after a stroke

Aphasia, the loss of language, is just one of the communication impairments that can be part of the clinical picture following a stroke and occurs in about a third of all cases. Also encountered are voice problems: dysphonia, articulation problems; dysarthria and perhaps motor programming problems for speech, and dyspraxia. Co-existing with these communication problems – and often the first reason an individual who has had a stroke meets a speech and language therapist – may be a swallowing problem, dysphagia. In addition there's an often overlooked area of communication problems associated with a right hemisphere stroke, e.g. problems understanding the more subtle complexities of communication such as inferred meaning. Where aphasia is the result of a stroke (i.e. not as a result of transient ischaemic attack, head injury, progressive neurological condition or infection such as encephalitis), the estimated incidence and prevalence for aphasia in a population of 100,000 is shown below (see refs. 2 & 3). As the prevalence figures are greater than the incidence of aphasia it goes without saying that many people who experience aphasia will require ongoing support and assistance, sometimes for years after the initial stroke.

Incidence	Prevalence		
per 100,000	per 100,000 of the population at any given time		
	moderate disability	*severe/chronic disability*	*total*
66	70	80	150

Services for people with aphasia

So, what support and services might be available if you experience communication or swallowing problems following a stroke? Whatever is written here will not reflect individual experience nor will it constitute a directory of services that will, should, or need to be provided. Each individual's needs will vary greatly. Additionally there is geographical variation in provision and there will be variation in individual clinicians: experience, creativity, area of special interest and philosophy. That said the Royal College of Speech and Language Therapists has been proactive in the introduction of professional standards and clinical guidelines to ensure best practice throughout the profession. Speech and language therapists working in the National Health Service are required to be registered members of the Royal College of Speech and Language Therapists. To re-register each year the therapist is required to complete a certain amount of continuing professional development, a written record of which must be witnessed by a fellow member. Perhaps most reassuring is that the field of aphasiology is an area rich with both clinical and academic researchers, employing both quantitative and qualitative methodologies to evaluate therapeutic interventions. Treatment efficacy has been widely demonstrated in specific impairments: the ability to communicate in everyday situations and, more broadly, in terms of social, emotional and psychological well-being.

The increased involvement seen in the 1980s and 1990s of the speech and language therapy profession in the assessment and management of swallowing problems put a strain on departmental resources. Many in the profession feared that the 'quality of life' communication work became a less pressing priority than the 'life and death' of swallowing problems. In an acute hospital environment speech and language therapists contribute much to improving the quality of people's lives following strokes by assessing and treating swallowing disorders. Such expertise will certainly have saved many from the misery and risks of aspiration pneumonia.

In hospitals where there is an established speech and language therapy department ward staff will know how to get the therapist along to see someone in their care. Even so it is worth knowing that speech and language therapy operates an open referral system, i.e. anyone can make a referral – professional, relative or the individual seeking assistance. The only exception to this will be where a swallowing assessment is required. The potential impact on medical condition of assessment and intervention for swallowing necessitates a doctor's referral. Bedside assessment is often the first contact and will involve, though not necessarily all in one go, a screening of communication problems, advice to facilitate communication on the ward, an invitation to family/next of kin to contact the speech and language therapist if they were not seen on the ward, information about communication problems and other useful organisations, e.g. Speakability, Connect, The Stroke Association or Headway, (see useful organisations on page 104). The advice at this stage can seem like a lot of common sense, coupled with a fair amount of reluctance (from the therapist) to respond definitively to questions about longer term outcome and ultimate recovery of speech. It's easy to forget just how complicated the human language is! In speaking, words come and go in fractions of seconds. For the normal listener, with language processing intact, each snippet of sound is speedily processed and a system of prediction about what will come next or what is required next will be operating, based on the listener's sophisticated knowledge of normal language. The following illustration is striking in speech but it works reasonably in writing too: If you hear someone say 'She used the knife to...' the listener just can't help a word popping into her head to fill the gap, e.g. cut or spread, etc. In contrast consider this example: Her husband rolled in drunk again and in a fit of rage she used the knife to...' and a different word may spring to mind. If a normal language user can be this sophisticated at such a small scale the language patterns observed in aphasia seem a little less mysterious. It becomes possible to imagine that there need only be a minor hiccup in language processing to derail the system spectacularly and, of course, following a stroke there's very likely been a more major derailment.

What happens beyond the acute hospital varies from service

to service. It may include regular therapy, review, an invitation to contact the department if problems persist or an out-patient appointment on discharge from the hospital. For some, once medically stable, there may be a period of further in-patient rehabilitation at a specialist stroke or neurorehabilitation unit. In general this occurs where the individual is experiencing more extensive or complex physical, cognitive and communication disability, requiring multidisciplinary management.

Theoretical influences on therapy approaches

Aphasiology is an area rich with the highest level of clinical and academic interest. The multidisciplinary membership of organisations such as the British Aphasiology Society, (see useful organisations on page 104), are evidence of this. As a result aphasia therapy is underpinned by extensive research and founded in recognised and developed theories of language processing and communicative behaviour.

WHO classifications

Like all rehabilitation professionals the speech and language therapist will be mindful of the World Health Organisation classifications of Impairment, Activity and Participation (see ref 4). Do these classifications matter in speech and language therapy intervention and what do they mean? A good illustration in communication terms would be where the impairment was one of inability to spell exceptional words, i.e. those that do not conform to normal spelling rules. The impact on activity might be that the person's writing is littered with regularised spelling mistakes and might be equivalent for people with similar levels of impairment. However the effect on a given individual's participation will vary according to the individual's need to be able to spell such words accurately. For example, the impact on participation for persons who make their living as proof readers will be much greater than the impact for persons who work as waiters. The table on page 99 illustrates this further.

Approaches to assessment and subsequent interventions initiated by speech and language therapists have developed and continue to develop, in these three areas.

Addressing impairments

Impairment level approaches underwent major revision in the 1980s and 1990s as cognitive neuropsychological theories of language processing and breakdown began to influence clinicians. A more problem-solving approach to communication problems following a stroke or other brain injury developed and, together with other theoretically motivated approaches addressing the impairment level there is now substantial evidence to suggest that aphasia therapy is efficacious (see refs. 5, 6, & 7). Furthermore, specific clinical assessment tools have been developed to assess impairment (see refs. 8 & 9). The impairment level approaches are sometimes accused of having little functional relevance, i.e. little to offer at an activity or participative level. However, the theoretically driven impairment approaches do enable therapists to apply 'hosepipe theory' to aphasia, i.e. if there's no water coming out of the hose it could be for any number of reasons – the tap is not on, there's a perforation in the hose, there's a kink in the hose, the water supply has been cut off, etc. Every cause produces the same effect but requires a different approach to resolve. Similarly, using a cognitive neuropsychological perspective to illustrate, the inability to name an object can be the result of a breakdown at differing language processing levels such as word meanings (semantics), word sounds (phonology), short term storage or articulation. As for the view that impairment therapies do not address the functional impact of the language disorder for the individual, creative clinicians strive to make even the simplest semantic (word meaning) therapy task functionally relevant by,

Problems (impairments)	Impact of problems on daily life (activity/participation)
Difficulty understanding simple spoken sentences	Cannot follow conversations Often chooses the wrong drink when offered a selection Only follows simple one-to-one conversation Cannot enjoy television/radio
Word finding problem	Limited participation in conversation Difficulty telling people how she/he is feeling Relies on partner to finish sentences Unable to use telephone effectively
Difficulty spelling exceptional/ irregular words	Slower writing letters College assignments have increased spelling errors Unable to keep up with note keeping in meetings/lectures
Poor self-monitoring	Doesn't notice when the words she/he produces are mispronounced Doesn't notice when she/he says the wrong word Is unaware she/he has difficulty understanding Doesn't recognise listeners' difficulty understanding him/her
Reading comprehension poor for complex syntactic structures	Unable to follow recipes Misunderstands official correspondence Requires assistance to manage personal correspondence

for example, using words or other stimuli that have functional relevance to a given individual. In so doing the clinician will also counter concern about item-specific improvement or carry-over to non-treated items. Furthermore, theoretical models of language processing can serve to provide some order and rationale for the chaotic speech, writing or comprehension patterns that form the surface and lay perception of aphasia. Interestingly, models of language processing are now an integral part of research into the functional neuroanatomy of communication, i.e. which bits of the brain do the processing necessary for communication (see ref. 10) and are being computer-tested both as models of normal function and to explore whether, when lesioned, these theoretical models produce impaired performance analogous to aphasic patterns (see ref. 11). What is not conclusively known, as yet, is whether there is a critical time for aphasia therapy to be effective. There is some suggestion that therapeutic intervention needs to be reasonably intensive, perhaps five hours per week. While assessment and the development and evaluation of therapeutic programmes would require a trained therapist, the daily practice could take the form of independent work or work with an appropriately briefed professional or lay person such as a healthcare assistant, volunteer or family member. Of course, professionals and loved ones need to be mindful that, while for some such roles can be a positive and empowering experience, for others it can be a tense, negative and destructive activity.

Looking beyond impairment

Speech and language therapy for aphasia is not solely about restoration of linguistic or cognitive function. At an early stage there should be some consideration of facilitating the individual's immediate communication needs. It cannot be assumed, although professionals and families often do, that the person with aphasia will be able to write or read instead of speaking. Perhaps even more surprising is that a person experiencing aphasia may not be able to use gesture to communicate either. Even those individuals with the physical, motor ability to make gestures may need encouragement and facilitation to recognise that such gestural skills can be used communicatively. It does not follow that a person with some understanding of single written words will be able to point to written words to convey messages or use a sophisticated, technologically advanced communication aid (see ref. 12). Conversely, assessment may reveal some intact processing which may be employed almost un-facilitated as an effective compensatory strategy (see ref. 13). So aphasia can involve the breakdown of the diverse aspects of symbolism and processing that form human communication in unexpected and surprising ways. Skilled speech and language therapy assessment will identify processes which may be employed successfully to facilitate communication. At this point the two-way nature of communication needs to be acknowledged and within the field of aphasia therapy there is increasing work encouraging the development and training of conversation partners for people with communication problems (see ref. 14), perhaps in tandem with specific linguistic therapy.

Psychosocial and emotional well-being

Inevitably there is a psychosocial and emotional impact of aphasia for the individual and those around him/her. The need to acknowledge, explore and provide support in this respect has always been recognised by the speech and language therapy profession. Furthermore, at Connect, for example, a counselling service is offered by trained counsellors with personal experience of aphasia.

Living with aphasia

Earlier in this chapter the more enduring nature of aphasia was alluded to in considering the prevalence figures. Perhaps, because speech and language therapy has developed pre-dominately within a medicine-led health service, the longer term needs have received less attention until recently. Hard-pressed health resources have focused on timely discharge. The speech and language therapy profession has always brought wide ranging skills to the support of all people with communication problems and openly and actively included families and carers in rehabilitation programmes. The long term impact of aphasia for individuals and those around them is now becoming a central area of the interest for clinical and research aphasiologists alike (see ref. 15). Research in this domain embraces social models of disability and qualitative research methodologies, such as ethnography. These extensive and varied approaches generally look beyond the linguistic though some, such as the training of conversation partners, represent a marriage of applied clinical linguistics and social facilitation (see ref. 16). Importantly there has been a move to develop aphasia-friendly resources (see ref. 17) and to include people with aphasia in the planning and development of services.

In summary, aphasia is as varied as it is complex. The assessment and treatment require methodical, creative, inclusive and empathetic approaches ranging from common sense advice to complex psycholinguistic programmes of therapy. Encouragingly, the wealth of published research in aphasiology suggests speech and language therapy is effective and professional support for the person with aphasia should always form part of the multidisciplinary network required for the effective delivery of a service to the survivors of strokes.

References

1   Parr S, Byng S, Gilpin S and Ireland C. *Talking about Aphasia: Living with Language Loss after Stroke*, OUP, 1997.

2   Enderby P and Phillip R. 'Speech and Language Handicap: Towards knowing the size of the problem', *British Journal of Disorders of Communication*, 1986, 21 (2), pp. 151–65.

3   Enderby P and Davies P. 'Communication disorders: Planning a service to meet the needs', *British Journal of Disorders of Communication*, 1989, 24, pp. 301–31.

4   WHO-Disability Functioning ICIDH-2 International classification of impairments, activities and participation.

5   Byng S. 'Hypothesis Testing and Aphasia Therapy', in Holland A and Forbes M (Eds), *Aphasia Treatment – World Perspectives*, 1993, San Diego: Singular, pp. 115–30.

6   Harding D and Pound C. 'Needs, Function and Measurement: Juggling with multiple language impairment', in Byng S, Swinburn K and Pound C, (Eds), *The Aphasia Therapy File*, Hove: Psychology Press, 1999.

7   Nickels L and Best W. 'Therapy for naming disorders (Part I): principles, puzzles and progress', *Aphasiology*, 1996, 10 (1), pp. 21–47.

     Nickels L and Best W. 'Therapy for naming disorders (Part I): specifics, surprises and suggestions', *Aphasiology*, 1996, 10 (2), pp. 109–36.

8   Kay J, Lesser R, and Coltheart M. *Psycholoinguistic assessments of language processing in aphasia*. Hove, UK: Psychology Press, 1992.

9   Whitworth A, Perkins L, and Lesser R. *Conversation analysis profile for people with aphasia*. London: Whurr, 1997.

10   Wise R J S, Scott S K, Blank S C, Mummery C J, Murphy K, and Warburton E A. 'Separate Neural Sub-systems within "Wernicke's Area" ', *Brain*, 2001, 124, pp. 83–95.

11   Martin N and Saffran E M. 'A computational account of deep dysphasia', *Brain and Language*, 1992, 43, pp. 240–274.

12 Harding D and Pound C. 'Needs, Function and Measurement: Juggling with multiple language impairment'. In Byng S, Swinburn K and Pound C, (Eds), *The Aphasia Therapy File*, Hove: Psychology Press, 1999.

13 Howard D and Harding D. 'Self-cueing of word retrieval by a woman with aphasia: why a letter board works', *Aphasiology*, 1998, 12 (4/5), pp. 399–420.

14 Kagan A. 'Supported conversation for adults with aphasia: methods and resources for training conversation partners', *Aphasiology*, 1998,12 (9), pp. 816–830.

15 Pound C, Parr S, Lindsay J and Woolf C. 'Beyond Aphasia', *Therapies for Living with Communication Disability*, London: Winslow, 2000.

16 Lock S, Wilkinson R and Bryan K. 'Supporting Partners of People with Aphasia'. *In Relationships and Conversations* (SPPARC), London: Winslow 2001.

17 Parr S, Pound C, Byng S and Long B. *The Aphasia Handbook*, Ecodistribution, Leicestershire, 1999.

Useful organisations

CONNECT — The communication disability network
16–18 Marshalsea Street
London SE1 1HL
Tel: 020 7367 0840

THE STROKE ASSOCIATION — Stroke House, Whitecross Street
London EC1Y 8JJ
Tel: 020 7490 7999

SPEAKABILITY — 1 Royal Street, London SE1 7LL
Tel: 020 7261 9572

HEADWAY — National Head Injuries Association
4 King Edward Court, King Edward Street
Nottingham NG1 1EW
Tel: 0115 924 0800

THE BRITISH APHASIOLOGY SOCIETY www.bas.org.uk

11

Neuroplasticity & the ARNI Approach to Functional Recovery from Stroke

TOM BALCHIN

IN 1997, at 21, I had an aneurysm followed by a subarachnoid haemorrhage which paralysed the left side of my body. My operation involved a craniotomy and clipping. Subarachnoid haemorrhage patients usually have a much longer recovery time than unruptured aneurysm patients, as well as more serious deficits than any other type of stroke. I was luckier than most. I personally made a good recovery because I researched, investigated and evaluated all the known techniques and strategies in as many physical arenas which could possibly have been of use to me to adapt and use to my own stroke survivor ends.

I spent years acquiring the necessary knowledge to re-habilitate myself and cope with life again. I worked out my own rehabilitative methods by becoming a strength athlete and martial arts expert, achieving the grade of 3rd Dan in Taekwondo whilst coping with one-sided weakness including drop-foot. I attained a Masters degree and a Doctorate before I was 30 years old. I also taught in schools and universities and developed a strong interest in researching giftedness and the creative brain.

A year after my stroke I was approached by other UK stroke survivors with requests for help to regain their movement and strength via my methods. And so, after doing more and more training of others in their houses and then running groups in local sports centres from 1998 to 2000, I decided to form ARNI (Action for Rehabilitation from Neurological Injury) in order to help stroke survivors in a structured way. My idea was to try and ensure that there is an increasing body of professional exercise instructors available to whom therapists (and other healthcare professionals) could feel comfortable about referring directly. We now have a charity, the ARNI Trust, which has over 80 highly qualified professional trainers around the UK, trained via our dedicated Functional Training After Stroke Accreditation (Middlesex University). Last year we estimated that since we started, over 6,000 stroke survivors had been trained in the ARNI Approach in one-to-one classes, massed practice sessions and shorter group classes.

Action for rehabilitation from neurological injury

ARNI is used by stroke networks, councils and stroke charities around the UK to train professional trainers. A more seamless care-pathway is the ideal. Stroke survivors around the country, upon application to the Trust, are matched up with qualified instructors. The goal is to retrain stroke survivors to a stage where successful vocational rehabilitation or community integration can occur. By 'retrain' we mean to help them work on their 'edges of current limitations', empower them to take controlled risks leading to success… and be creative with their own recoveries. The idea is to take stroke survivors back to (if required) a functional standard that they were left in after therapy input, and then go further than the standard that the hospitals had the time, resources or workable strategies to deliver to them.

The value-added of using professional exercise instructors is that the functional retraining they are tasked to deliver is an obvious way to seek to prevent expensive long-term re-hospitalisation, due to decline after therapy or injury via attempted risk-taking. For example, at Chaul End Day Centre in

Luton, audit data reported 24 ambulance calls out over one year to help clients who had fallen over. In the year after, when the Centre offered a one hour class plus a drop-in facility run by three ARNI Instructors, there were no call outs at all, with a direct ambulance service saving of £7,200. This was because patients dramatically reduced their frequency of falling and learned how to get up *themselves, without support* if they did. This latter strategy is a 'signature' ARNI strategy, called the 'Gatekeeper' and is itself the subject of a current clinical research proposal.

The clinical effectiveness and cost effectiveness of the ARNI Approach was the focus of an application for a national multi-centre RCT (£2.1 million) in June 2010 by the Peninsula Collaboration for Leadership in Applied Health Research and Care (PenCLAHRC) and the South West Stroke Research Network (SWSRN). This is called the ReTrain Project. Other research from 2010 to 2011 included a 48-week feasibility study by Brunel University using four groups of stroke survivors (n=36), referred to the ARNI training programme by Hillingdon Hospital, UK.

Because ARNI strategies are being shown anecdotally time and time again to have clearly positive results with stroke and ABI survivors around the UK in terms of tackling action control, strength and confidence issues, NHS Stroke Network representatives, clinicians, hospital directors and therapists working in the areas of neurorehabilitation have actively recognised and encouraged its efforts for some time. ARNI has won formal recognition for its originality in the field. For example, in November 2010, at the first United Kingdom Acquired Brain Injury Forum Awards in London, ARNI was considered by the judges to have shown '*the best example of innovation by a voluntary sector provider or registered charity in the field of ABI*'.

The ARNI approach

The ARNI Approach is a manual-based rehabilitation pro-gramme, constructed around current evidence-based neuro-logical research perspectives. ARNI instructors either visit trainees' houses or meet them in gyms to train them on a one-to-one basis. Some also run dedicated stroke groups, often with the help of other instructors or assistants who can support the initiation of the kind of functional training. The ARNI approach is very successful in terms of offering options for real self-recovery and self-management of the physical limitations caused by stroke. It highlights autonomy (or supported autonomy) over training efforts. This is a major goal that instructors are required to promote.

The role of the trainer is seen as a respected health and fitness professional who is one step removed from the hospitals or other physiotherapy setting. This is vital in order to further re-integrate patients to society, normalise them and facilitate them to take charge. The trainer nurtures and supports the individual's drive to physical recovery in a one-to-one situation or within a group class, and guides them into a pattern of self-reliance.

The strategies, stretches and exercises must make sense to the trainee. The trainee must try hard to repeat and innovate upon the whole tasks they have worked on in class, repeatable when class is finished, as 'homework'. The idea is to enthuse and arm stroke survivors with know-how, concerning 'what they need to do next to progress', and to support a positive and upward slope to success in terms of increased robusticity, action control and strength.

The ARNI Approach uses short, formal training and massed practice sessions which encompass task-related training, physical coping strategies and resistance training. All of these three complement each other and the sum of the three have been shown to give better outcomes from the limitations from stroke than using them separately. The Approach was grown over using these three principles combined with hard work and motivational boosting as its fundamental tenet. Moreover, as the years go by, more and more evidence is emerging that it is correct to be using such an approach to recovery from stroke. For example, Dutch researchers in 2006 reviewed all available published clinical stroke rehabilitation trials, of which at the time of writing there existed 735. They selected 151 studies including 123 randomised controlled trials and 28 controlled trials. In their consideration, the rest either did not meet the inclusion criteria or lacked statistical and internal validity, reflecting the poor methodological quality of many clinical intervention studies.

The Dutch researchers found that traditional treatment approaches induce improvements that are confined to impairment level only and *do not generalise to a functional improvement level.* In contrast, they concluded that evidence existed that: *'more recently developed treatment strategies that incorporate compensation strategies with a strong emphasis on functional training, may hold the key to optimal stroke rehabilitation'.* In summing up their findings, they reported that *'intensity and task-specific exercise therapy are important components of such an approach'.*

I have found that there is a strong case for implementing and balancing both into an Approach, with the addition of strength training. It's what I did instinctively (and still do) to retrain, manage and 'negate' my own physical limitations. The Approach suggests that during activities of daily life, the lessons learned from formal retraining (two to three times per week) must be introduced, practised and trialled safely when performing activities of daily life (all the time). Formal retraining aims to give a safe arena in which to practise for the expected and the unexpected.

Similarly, the training can sustain and make available vital extra interventions such as CIMT, EMG biofeedback, FES, inter-active robotic therapy, interactive metronome, virtual reality training, etc. All require task-related training of some sort, either as part of the intervention or afterwards. BOTOX too, requires a post-injection retraining programme to be in place. The Approach recognises that clients will be looking at treatment options to heighten the effects of rehabilitation. For instance FES, combined with rehabilitation enhanced plastic reorganisation of the affected motor cortex, has been shown to lead to superior behavioural recovery. Clearly, whatever the physiological mechanism underpinning, if the technique doesn't enable the individual to achieve the goals in the expected timeframe then another intervention is needed. The Approach aims to be a constant within which the patient can explore the effects of extraneous interventions which concur with the principles of neuroplasticity.

Neuroplasticity

Neuroplasticity is very good news. It is the saving grace of the damaged brain. Without it, lost functions to a large extent could never be regained, nor could disabled processes ever hope to be improved. The brain consists of nerve cells (or 'neurons') and glial cells which are interconnected. They transmit messages via electrochemical impulses. Neuroplasticity (also referred to as brain plasticity, cortical plasticity or cortical re-mapping) is the *changing* of these neurons, the organisation of their networks, and their functions via new experiences.

After an injury to the cerebral cortex, the structure and function of sensory and motor regions are drastically altered. A loss of fine motor control and the employment of compensatory movement strategies is normally the result. However, the surviving brain tissue may be substantially altered in its basic anatomic connectivity. Neuroplasticity, in effect, involves changes in the strength of the connections, by adding or removing connections (recruiting nearby connections to gradually take over the 'lost' movement), or by adding new cells.

All the thinking, learning, and activities a survivor attempts to do after a stroke will inform and physically change both their brain's structure (anatomy) and functional organisation (physiology) from top to bottom.

The very idea of the brain being able to 'adapt' to a traumatic event is one of the most extraordinary discoveries of the twentieth century. Irrefutable evidence has been found that the brain can substantially reorganise itself in response to the input it is, or is not, receiving after stroke. Basically, the brain appears to have the ability to seek out older, less-used roads if the 'main road' is blocked. Neuroplasticity allows us to compensate for irreparably damaged neural pathways by strengthening or rerouting remaining ones.

No two brains are the same. Your brain, even if you had never had a stroke, is very different from your friend's brain. It is wired uniquely. The differences relate mainly to your life experiences and the things that you do. For instance, if you start playing the violin, juggling or learning a language, the structure of your brain itself will immediately change and perfect its circuitry to render the task in question.

How is this possible? Your amazing brain constructs different representations of space. It creates maps or 'schema' concerning its own shape and potential, guided by both sensory inputs (received from seeing, hearing and touching things) and motor output (signals to shape movements). It creates a spatial chart via the integration of different sensory and motor systems. This chart maps a representation of your own body (personal space), the space surrounding our bodies that can be reached by our limbs (peripersonal space) and space beyond the reach of our limbs (extrapersonal space). Peripersonal space is the distinct representation of the visual space about 30 cm around the upper body, particularly the hands and the feet.

These body maps are laid out in small strips and spread around different sections across the surface of your brain. They are profoundly adaptable and changeable. Amazingly, they are being updated all the time. The sensory map can for example, instantly expand and contract to include everyday objects. Healthy cells surrounding an injured area of your brain can change their function and even their shape, so as to perform the tasks and transfer signals previously dealt with by the now-damaged neurons at the site of injury. This process is called *functional map expansion.*

Because brain structures are dynamic and constantly remodelling in response to learning and experience, it is being revealed that *neuroplasticity is possible at any point following your stroke*, if specified conditions or meaningful and enriched environmental contexts are present during practice. *Task-related practice* is the number one way to retrain the brain. It means simply to train the action to be performed in a natural environment. Stroke survivors need to be *doing* the task they want to do. So, to practise for going up and down steps, you practise going up and down steps in a controlled environment.

Think of neuroplasticity as real-time changes taking place concerning the amount of brain surface area dedicated to sending and receiving signals from some specific part of the body. And the more habitually that you try to use a particular movement (and indeed voluntarily, rather than being 'forced' to), the more 'real estate' becomes devoted to that particular muscle group to compose that movement. Positive synaptic rewiring (functional connections between neurons) can take place very quickly.

Now there is evidence that your brain is able to recruit remaining neural networks (usually near the lesion) to perform the similar functions of the damaged ones. Sometimes this even includes networks in areas of your brain that were not normally involved in the specific motor system. Neuroplasticity needs very specific input with the proper stimulus which should be done regularly enough to become a habit. The stroke survivor is encouraged to try to do something new with his or her affected limb by themselves each day. Repeated attempts to use affected limbs in training creates a form of practice that can potentially lead to further improvement in performance. A 'virtuous circle', can be entered into in which spontaneous limb use and motor performance will reinforce each other and re-teach the body to control the position of an affected limb.

All rehabilitation needs to attend to specific functional goals. The ARNI Approach recommends that in formal retraining situations it is important to advance quickly toward practice of whole tasks with as much of the *environment context* made available as possible. For example, say, a goal of the discharged survivor has been identified to be a desire to improve the action control of their paretic foot for being able to cope whilst walking outside, unsupervised and with no supports. The best retraining he or she can get is to ask a trainer or friend to plan a route for them to go with him or her, so that they can trial it safely and under careful supervision. They can work on leaving sticks or supports behind or using/wearing them according to their current levels of ability.

Stroke survivors ultimately seek spontaneous co-ordinated limb movement. Much of 'proprioception' (the sense of knowing where a body part is in space) occurs without conscious thought. An increase in motor performance resulting from reversal of the loss of representation of limbs in the brain after training is proposed to increase spontaneous use of limbs, as the brain takes more responsibility of muscle control.

Brains learn what they do. And for such adaptation to happen optimally, stroke survivors must be prepared to do some focused work with whatever movement they possess, even if you believe they have none at all. A phenomenal number of repetitions are posited to be required for optimal neural rewiring: over and over again, with as much attention to detail as can be mustered.

Using simultaneous movement of both limbs seems to work well for stroke. Just one way that this is done in the ARNI Approach that might be recognisable to readers is *bilateral movement training*: a concept based on the theory of inter-limb coordination. Cumulative evidence from a review of several studies that investigated results from bilateral movement training for partially paralysed upper body indicates that bilateral movement training is effective in improving motor capabilities and functional outcome in the sub-acute or chronic (six months or longer from stroke onset) phase of recovery.

Task variability is another element of the Approach. New studies, especially in the field of interactive computer gaming for stroke rehabilitation, are showing that introducing task variability (random practice) improves performance in subsequent sessions and is more effective than blocked repetition of a constant task. It may be that task-variability helps cortical representation very well. *We are talking about nothing less than 'directed neuroplasticity'; trying to impose sequences of input and specific repetitive patterns of stimulation in order to cause desirable and specific changes in the brain.* Imagining specific movements (e.g. mental movement therapy) and creating optimal experiences which strongly relate to the tasks they ultimately want to complete are keys to trigger neuroplastic change for which strong positive evidence now exists.

A caveat however is that the idea that recovery from stroke is 'all about neuroplasticity' may be too simplistic. It is important to appreciate that in some cases stroke damage may be so extensive and severe that remaining neural networks may be too weak to be 'retrained'.

There may have to be enough remaining neural networks to 're-programme' for plasticity to work although recent studies have suggested that long-range intra-cortical pathways can be rerouted to completely novel territories, not just those near to the lesion. This surprising ability of the cerebral cortex may yield important clues to improving functional recovery in stroke survivors by using retraining in a knowledgeable attempt to modulate post-injury anatomy in a more adaptive way.

References

1. Balchin, T. (2011).*The Successful Stroke Survivor*. Lingfield: Bagwin Press, pp. 15–54.

2. Kollen, B, Gert Kwakkel, G & Lindeman, E. (2006). Functional Recovery After Stroke: A Review of Current Developments in Stroke Rehabilitation Research. Reviews on Recent Clinical Trials, 2006, 1, 75–80.

3. Plautz E, Nudo R. (2005). Neural plasticity and functional recovery following cortical ischemic injury. Engineering in Medicine and Biology Society. EMBS '06. 27th Annual International Conference of the IEEE, 4:4145-8.

4. Nudo R, Barbay S, Kleim J. (2000) Role of neuroplasticity in functional recovery after stroke. In: Levin HS, Grafman J, eds. *Cerebral Reorganization of Function after Brain Damage*. Vol 1. USA: Oxford University Press; p. 168-197.

5. Draganski B, Gaser C, Busch V, Schuierer G, Bogdahn U, May A. (2004). Neuroplasticity: changes in grey matter induced by training. Nature 427(6972):311-2.

6. Schicke, T, Bauer, F, & Röder, B. (2009). Interactions of different body parts in peripersonal space: how vision of the foot influences tactile perception at the hand. Experimental Brain Research, 192, 4, pp. 703-715.

7. Kleim J, Jones T, Schallen T. (2003). Motor enrichment and the induction of plasticity before or after brain injury. Neurochem Research. 28:1757-1769.

8. Kolb, B. (2003). Overview of cortical plasticity and recovery from brain injury. Phys Med Rehabil Clin N Am. 14:S7-25, viii.

9. Szturm T, Peters JF, Otto C, Kapadia N, Desai, A. (2008). Task-specific rehabilitation of finger-hand function using interactive computer gaming. Arch Phys Med Rehabil; 89: 2213-7.

10. Nudo, R. (2007). Postinfarct Cortical Plasticity and Behavioral Recovery, Stroke. 38: 840-845.

12
Different doctors –
a personal view*

PROFESSOR D L MCLELLAN

DOCTORS TEND TO BE CRITICISED for focusing too much on diseases and not enough on the people who have them. Someone who experiences a stroke needs to be able to explore with their doctor not only what a stroke is, but how to understand and cope with the experience, and then how best to face the future. This means that doctors need to understand not only the medical aspects of stroke, but equally the turmoil experienced by the patient and family and the processes by which this turmoil can be worked through during rehabilitation.

This is a tall order for doctors and especially for young ones, most of whom have yet to experience in their own lives the upheaval of major life events. Many stroke patients have already experienced such life events and will certainly be experiencing one after their stroke. Yet it is junior hospital doctors who will be the first to see someone admitted to hospital after a stroke, and who will be the doctors most closely involved in their day-to-day experience when in hospital.

How do young doctors learn about the significance of stroke for a person's life story and sense of identity, without having to reach the same age and to have had the same experience as their patients? This is achieved partly through their formal education

---

*This article was first published in *Different Strokes*.

and training and crucially by the example of their 'role models', their consultants. If their consultants are seen to give priority to understanding what the stroke means to their patients and what their fears are, then junior doctors will seek to do the same and will value this expertise in themselves. If, however, the consultant appears to be interested only in the diagnostic aspects of the stroke, and the use of drugs to treat it, and if the main expectation placed on the junior doctor is simply to get the patient discharged from hospital as soon as humanly possible, then this inadequate agenda will tend to be passed on to the next generation of consultants and so the cycle will be repeated.

Understanding the experience of stroke, and recognising the need to provide better help, is one of the major aims of the speciality of rehabilitation medicine. Britain's newest speciality, it was formally established across the UK for the first time only in 1989. From a base of about 15 consultants and 4 trainees in 1989 it has developed to over 120 consultants and 45 trainees today, and these numbers are expanding as fast as young doctors can be attracted into the speciality. What is different about rehabilitation? Most NHS rehabilitation services are organised with older, retired people in mind. However, younger people have different agendas in their rehabilitation. Disabled school leavers may be seeking to establish themselves independently as young adults for the first time. A little later they will be grappling with the early stages of their adult careers, where the increasing demands of work and family will create different priorities. More intensive therapies and demanding treatments will be appropriate for younger people with greater physical energy, whose lives are still being carved out.

Young doctors training in rehabilitation medicine are taught the importance of understanding the meaning of stroke to younger individuals and families who experience one. They are taught that, while two strokes may appear much the same, two people with strokes never are and that the attributes and objectives of the person who has a stroke are crucial elements in negotiating what rehabilitation should aim at and what form it should take. To serve younger people in the UK effectively we need at least 250 consultants. We currently have 110. We need to get an equally strong commitment from social services, local councils, the voluntary sector and the employment and education services.

One of the challenges in rehabilitation generally is to promote areas of knowledge and the specific practices of each profession, at the same time as ensuring that they work together as members of a genuine rehabilitation team when they need to. When professions are young they tend to be unsure of their role and status and they are instinctively better at competing than at collaborating across boundaries. However, in the past 15 years there has been a transformation of the academic base of the therapy professions, who are now established in universities and who have increasingly adopted the university tradition of multi-disciplinary and inter-disciplinary research and training. Britain developed the world's first national multidisciplinary research society, the Society for Research into Rehabilitation, which rapidly grew into a thriving scientific body, with international links across the world. At Society of Rehabilitation meetings (the proceedings of which are regularly published in the scientific journal *Clinical Rehabilitation*), new research can be debated in a multi-professional setting.

Sounds very grand, doesn't it? But when will I see results (I hear you ask) in the behaviour of doctors in my local hospital, health centre or community NHS services? The answer is that you should be starting to see it already, especially if you have seen a consultant in rehabilitation medicine locally, or your doctor has been exposed to rehabilitation medicine during training. Our specialists are committed to working as closely as possible with the other rehabilitation professionals, and also with social and voluntary sector services. With them we are campaigning for unified management structures and budgets, and unified planning of development of services at each locality, in order to promote rehabilitation. Central to any such development is consumer involvement both in the planning and implementation of services. Organisations such as Different Strokes are very important players here.

The British Society of Rehabilitation Medicine is committed not only to improving specialist medical practice in rehabilitation, but to developing a fundamental concept in medical thinking and behaviour. Those shameful days when consultants on their 'rounds' would walk past stroke patients without even speaking to them should be a thing of the past but we recognise there is still a long way to go.

Part 3

STROKE AND DIFFERENT
AGE GROUPS:
CHILDREN, YOUNG ADULTS
AND THE ELDERLY

13
Different age groups

THE PUBLIC PERCEPTION of stroke is still that it only affects the elderly, but strokes can strike at any time of life. When it occurs to a young person or a child, the shock and disbelief is enormous. Information is hard to find, families feel isolated and, worse still, treatment and after care are often woefully inadequate or inappropriate.

Strokes and children

'Childhood stroke has been known for centuries. It is defined as any child between one month and sixteen years of age who has had a stroke. As in adults, there are many causes. Unlike adults, the number of children having strokes is unknown, but for the United Kingdom it is felt to be between 250 to 1000 cases per annum.'

This statement comes from the synopsis of the *National Childhood Stroke Study* (Dr A N Williams 1999). The statistics may come as a surprise to parents faced with their child who has had a stroke. To them it is a singular experience and they will feel bewildered. It is likely that they will have not heard of a previous case and will be desperate for information about how to proceed after the acute stage is over.

Priorities are very different for the three age groups. Leaving aside the medical aspects, children need to be able to get back to school and continue their education as soon as possible. They need their friends as well as the understanding of their teachers and education authorities for whatever support and assistance they may need. The time scale is so different. If a recovery, allowing an individual to take part in normal activities, takes a year or even two for someone much older, this might not be too serious – for a child this is a considerable period in their development. In education any period, once missed is hard to replace; even missing a term puts added strain as a pupil tries to catch up.

All ages of stroke patients tend to be left with some similar problems, but they may affect their daily life in slightly different ways. Take fatigue; it affects both performance and memory. A child may be competent at the beginning of the day – or week – and hardly remember a thing at the end. Will teachers understand? How accurate is an assessment taken at one extreme or another? Someone may appear to be competent when moving slowly and purposefully, but what happens when hurried? It is difficult to explain the upset that may occur when you are forced to try to perform any action at speed. Something like a fire practice at school, might induce real panic in a child. Particular worries are involved when changing from primary to secondary school. Will there be stairs without rails on both sides or even steps with no supports occasionally at the new site? Children hate to stand out as different – what will other children say? It is distressing to learn from parents how much some children worry about such things, even to the extent of not being able to sleep. Such tensions will affect all aspects of performance. There are commonsense solutions to many of these problems but how often are they dealt with in a sensitive way in an overstretched education system?

Echoing what Jane Cast said about adult patients needing help long after support had ceased (see page 68): child patients grow into adolescents with all the insecurities and problems involved. An emotional backlash would not be surprising as teenagers realise the implications of their condition. It would make little difference at that moment whether their worst fears were realistic or not, and a teenager might not be able or willing to voice them.

I would like to point out that what I have said on page 16 about handwriting, and what I recommend for adults may not necessarily be right for children. They need to be able to produce written work as soon as possible to keep up with their school work. Some children can adjust to using their non-preferred hand quite easily. One primary pupil I know developed an efficient writing quickly and found little difficulty in keeping up with his peers. Other children have lost the use of their non-preferred hand and so can still write, but there is a downside. In both circumstances I have noticed that the affected hand is not being used sufficiently (whether receiving therapy or not) to regain strength and usage without that motivation that the desire to write provides. The more the affected hand and arm are ignored the more one-sided the child will become or have other problems (see page 19).

One parent distinctly remembers a doctor saying that she should 'write off' her child's preferred hand as useless and concentrate on retraining the non-preferred one. By the time this was achieved and the implications realised she reported that it was too late, too tiring and dispiriting to do much about the situation. Everyone needs two efficient hands if possible, so a balanced attitude is desirable towards encouraging gradual and appropriate use of the preferred hand, but admittedly that balance is not easy to achieve.

An American friend sent me this apt quote that she found on an OT website: 'I have a four-year-old girl on my caseload who has right-side post-stroke involvement. One day she just came out and told me her hand doesn't work. I told her she's got to tell it to work better or it won't know. Well, she started saying to her hand, "Hand, work better!" and it did.' What an excellent way of explaining to a young child just what we adults usually have to find out for ourselves. Older patients should learn from this simple statement, because, believe me, telling your hand or foot what to do is exactly what you may need to do for quite some while before it learns to perform a certain action by itself.

My correspondent conjectured whether small children were better at 'mind over matter' than older people. It is that clear explanation that works whatever the age and it is wrong to suppose that young children are any less motivated to help themselves than someone older, once they are pointed in the right direction. There is another factor to consider. Child patients are not unintelligent and should be listened to, just like adults. Therapists are not invariably right. For instance, when prescribing aids – children may be able to feel what suits their body or meets their needs and what does not. Anyhow they are unlikely to make full use of something when they are not comfortable with it.

As a family, we learned a lot when our youngest daughter, then aged six, suffered a sudden, serious neurological condition not dissimilar to a stroke. Something like this affects the whole family. Parents' lives are obviously disrupted as they have to alter priorities, but what about siblings? They also suffer as their activities may be severely curtailed. Their own feelings can vary from acute distress to the perhaps more natural angry reaction for a young child of: 'Why should this happen to us. It's not fair'. It may be difficult for them to understand, however hard parents may try, why most of the focus must now be on the patient and his or her needs. This may have to be the case for many months, even years, creating real hardship. On the other hand it can unite everyone and strengthen family ties.

Attitudes of those around them affect young patients too. I wonder now how my own worries added to my daughter's so I asked her, 25 years later, what she remembered. She recalled that she was hypersensitive to hushed tones and funny looks. She was able to see through what she called doctors' and nurses' false cheerfulness and could tell when things were going wrong. 'Children tune in to body language', she says.

I will never forget the consultant who voiced a dire prognosis in front of my child. She revealed, by occasional comments, how well she had understood and how it preyed on her mind for several years before it became obvious that what was prophesied was not going to happen. We survived the first difficult year because we had the help of a wise paediatrician locally (the late Dr Peter Swift). There are, however, many positive factors to give parents hope. Children who go through such experiences become exceptionally motivated teenagers and sensitive, caring adults. They frequently overcome their difficulties in the end and delight in proving the experts wrong.

Across the country many parents of children recovering from a stroke feel isolated. They tell me that they deplore the lack of a network and helpline for parents. They stress the need for user-friendly leaflets (in different languages), preferably written by parents who have experience. They plead for a support group like Different Strokes, specially for parents of young child patients.

Dr Fenella Kirkham is a paediatric neurologist based at the Institute of Child Health and at Southampton General Hospital. She has a special interest in child stroke patients and has contributed a chapter, from the perspective of a consultant, outlining the possible causes, necessary investigations and likely treatments for a child with a stroke. She emphasises how families can help their own children, all of which is particularly valuable as the subject is so little understood. To have access to such information is important for all concerned with the care and guidance of children

Young adults

Each year over 10,000 people of working age in the UK have a stroke. Over 1000 of them are under the age of 30, reports the organisation Different Strokes. The following quotation comes from a summary of *A Study to Evaluate the Met and Unmet*

Needs of Young Stroke Survivors, by D L McLellan, P Kersten, A Ashburn and A George:

> 'Although stroke is the most common cause of adult disability in the UK there is a lack of knowledge about an individual's perception of their own recovery. There is evidence to show that organised services for people with stroke can help to increase independence. There are also some indications that the needs of people who have had a stroke, and their carers are inadequately met.'

Many young stroke survivors would, I am sure, echo the last sentence. For young adults the main concern might be how they will be able to get back to work or their studies and support themselves and their families, as well as to live a full life in other ways. Being aware of the implications, and devastating effect on them and all around them, and yet with their whole lives before them, young stroke survivors deserve the very best treatment – but are they getting it? They have a champion in Donal O'Kelly. He was a barrister of twenty years, specialising in criminal and family law, who suffered a severe, brain stem stroke when in court. Because of the inadequacy in the system that he and other fellow stroke sufferers experienced he founded Different Strokes to cater for the needs of young adults and those up to the age of fifty-five.

The annual conference of this organisation in 2000 gave a good idea of its various functions. First, there was a presentation on cognitive rehabilitation, by Kit Malia. He defined cognition as: 'The working of the mind through which we make sense of the world'. He analysed the various components under five headings: attention, visual processing, information processing, memory and executive problems. He then enlarged on each of these to show how a stroke might affect any aspect of cognition. A progress report on the research project 'Work after Stroke' followed. There were also practical workshops, and the audience were just as interesting as the speakers. Many people spoke of the support and comradeship they found in the exercise groups. A lady explained how she had heard of the work that Salisbury was doing (see page 72) through the Different Strokes' newsletter and already had an ODFS to help her walk. Now, five years on from her stroke, she was embarking on a device to help her non-functional arm and hand – having had no treatment for them in the intervening years. As she said: '... it is only the positive ones like us who get to meetings like this' – we ought to worry about the rest. There were also therapists and researchers, including the team from Glasgow involved in the research study into the needs of younger stroke survivors and their families (see page 156). I got the impression that treatment in Scotland was better than in England. Anyone attending the conference could learn a lot about what can be done for stroke, what is being done and what still needs to be done.

The elderly

In March 2001 the Department of Health published the National Service Framework (NSF) for Older People. To coincide with this the Stroke Association commissioned the College of Health to carry out a large survey of stroke patients and carers. Their findings are reported in Speaking out about Stroke Services. Replies to their questionnaire highlighted considerable variability in the perceptions of care available. This report makes disconcerting reading, especially after the previous Stroke Association's report in 1999, *Stroke Care – A Matter of Chance* (see also page 22), following another in 1992. Together they illustrate the lamentably slow rate of improvement in services for the elderly. Perhaps it is misleading to quote only negative comments, but they are most relevant to this age group:

(1) 'I was told by the consultant that my husband was geriatric and therefore did not qualify for intensive therapy.'

(2) 'I'm afraid to say I think I was written off and forgotten.'

(3) 'God help old people on their own with no-one to fight their corner – and believe me fight is the appropriate word.'

Carers also voiced their concerns but, apart from the medical and support needs, what are the priorities for elderly patients? For those, particularly those who live alone, the primary concern will be with mobility and safety. The question always in their minds and those of their families will be whether they will be able to continue with independent living. What help will be available once they are discharged and how will they and their partners – if any – manage?

Together with my contributions as an elderly stroke survivor and the other contributors to this section a wide perspective is given to the problems of the different age groups. If I had anything to add it would be to say that whatever the age, health professionals (and carers) should try to project themselves into the mind of the patient. They must try to feel what it is like to be them as they struggle to come to terms with their condition in their particular environment.

14
Strokes in childhood

DR FENELLA KIRKHAM

S̶TROKE CONTINUES to be an important problem in children, affecting at least as many as brain tumour, although with considerably less media attention and health service resources. The perception that nothing can be done is now changing and it is likely that stroke services for young people in general, and children in particular, will improve, so that all can benefit from the ongoing scientific and technological advances. This article outlines the possible causes, necessary investigations and likely treatments for a child with a stroke and emphasises how families can help their own children.

Causes

One of the problems is that there is a very long list of possible causes of stroke, which both doctors and families find very daunting. In fact, most of these are very rare and at least half of children with stroke present 'out-of-the-blue', having never been seriously ill before. World-wide, the commonest cause is sickle cell disease, and in this condition stroke is as common in mid-childhood as it is in elderly adults in general. Cardiac disease is another important cause, although the proportion of children affected has probably fallen as curative surgery has been performed at younger and younger ages, since the risk is almost always reduced after successful operation.

The main thrust of the current research concerns the cause of stroke in the children for whom it occurs 'out-of-the-blue'. Occasionally a clot may arise from the heart, but this is probably less common than in adults with stroke. Minor injury plays a part in some. There is increasing evidence that infection, e.g. recent chickenpox and recurrent tonsilitis, plays a role; but of course, most children who catch these relatively minor illnesses don't have a stroke. It is likely that those who do, have a predisposition, perhaps genetic, to developing blood vessel narrowing and obstruction when triggered by a common infection. Predispositions might include a tendency to clot more easily or to damage and/or repair the blood vessel much more than average. If the blood vessel wall is narrowed, then a stroke may not happen unless brain tissue is short of oxygen, for example if there is anaemia secondary to iron deficiency or sickle cell disease or hypoxia in a child who is 'blue' because of heart disease or has upper airway obstruction overnight. It is likely that a child with stroke has a combination of risk factors, including a recent trigger, such as trauma or infection, a tendency to relatively sticky blood and some reason for a slightly reduced oxygen supply to the brain tissue.

Tests

When a child presents with acute weakness of one side, one of the first priorities is to establish whether or not there has been bleeding into the brain, which might need surgical removal. CT scanning is a very good method of doing this, although it is not so good at showing if there has been a clot in an artery causing a lack of blood supply to an area of brain (ischaemic stroke), particularly if this is small or if the scan is performed within 24 hours. MRI is better at demonstrating ischaemic stroke, and has the added advantage of being able to show the arteries and veins inside the head. It is now possible to show areas of brain where the blood flow is low but the brain is not yet damaged, and occasionally areas of brain which are very short of oxygen but still capable of surviving. Usually, there is enough information from either a CT or an MRI scan, but occasionally other imaging may be needed such as an arteriogram, a better method of showing the blood vessels, or a single photon emission computed tomography (SPECT) scan, which shows areas of reduced blood flow. The aim is to show whether there is an area of damage and, if so, where; whether there is an abnormality of the blood vessels and, if so, what type, and in some circumstances, whether there is an area of low cerebral blood flow beyond the area of damage.

An echocardiogram (ECHO) is usually performed, to see if there is any structural abnormality e.g. a small hole. A normal electrocardiogram (ECG) excludes the possibility of an abnormal rhythm, which can be associated with clots in the heart breaking off and migrating into the brain circulation, although this is rare in children. A lot of blood is taken, looking for evidence of infection or of a tendency to anaemia or increased blood stickiness or abnormally high lipid levels, e.g. cholesterol. Sometimes specific genetic testing is performed, e.g. for Factor V Leiden which is definitely associated with venous clotting in the legs. A chemical called homocysteine, which is associated with damage to the blood vessel wall if in high concentration, may be measured. Lumbar puncture is often performed, as meningitis is an important cause, and some children with recent chickenpox have abnormal spinal fluid. If there is a history of recurrent tonsillitis or snoring, children may have an overnight sleep study, where oxygen levels are measured, using a small skin probe.

Treatment

If the blood vessel is blocked, the brain tissue beyond it dies after about three hours. It has proved possible, in adults, to unblock the artery and save the brain tissue by using tissue plasminogen activator, but only within a three hour time window; beyond this

133

time there is a high risk of bleeding. It is exceptional for a child to be eligible for this sort of treatment, particularly as it is not appropriate for those who have recently had a procedure, i.e. the majority who stroke in hospital. Emergency transfusion is indicated for children with sickle cell disease who stroke. Occasionally, surgery may be needed, e.g. to remove a large amount of blood or damaged tissue pressing on the brain. For the majority of children, there is nothing that can be done to reduce the amount of damage done at the time of the first stroke and effort is concentrated on preventing further episodes.

Overall, the risk of further stroke is around 10 per cent, but is higher in some groups, e.g. those with sickle cell disease, and lower in others. There is some evidence that genetic predisposition, for example to high homocysteine levels which damage the blood vessel walls, may play a part in encouraging further episodes of blockage, usually in the same blood vessel, but occasionally in others. This is important, as homocysteine can be lowered by increasing the intake of B vitamins, particularly folic acid, vitamin B6 and vitamin B12. For some children, for example those with sickle cell disease, recurrent stroke appears to be related to anaemia and/or hypoxia. Blood transfusion has been seen to reduce the recurrence risk in this group and oxygen supplementation is under investigation. If the blood vessels are completely blocked, e.g. in Moyamoya (a Japanese term describing the puff of smoke appearance on the arteriogram of the collateral blood vessels attempting to bypass the blockage), then if the blood flow is low, it may be increased after bypass surgery to attach a scalp blood vessel to the blocked one.

Occasionally, it may be appropriate for a child to receive anticoagulation, for example if there is a genetic predisposition to increased blood stickiness, e.g. Factor V Leiden. However, there is a risk of bleeding and patients have to have frequent blood tests. In the majority of children with stroke 'out-of-the-blue', for whom no obvious cause has been found, low dose aspirin (1mg/kg) is prescribed in the medium term, as it has few risks and has been shown to reduce the risk of further strokes in adults. The only way of proving that a treatment is worth taking to reduce the risk of recurrence is to conduct a controlled trial with a large enough number of patients, randomly allocated to one treatment or another or to a placebo.

In addition to specific treatments, changes in lifestyle may reduce the risk of recurrence. It is certainly sensible to eat five portions of fruit or vegetables a day and to take plenty of exercise, e.g. walking to school. Every child should have a balanced diet, with fat and salt-laden foods, e.g. hamburgers and sausages, seen as occasional treats rather than staple foods.

Many children and their parents are devastated by the stroke and anxious about the future. These needs should be met by appropriate professional and lay support.

Making progress

Although many children have a severe weakness of the affected arm and leg immediately after the stroke, the majority make a good recovery and almost all walk, usually with only a minimal limp. Early physiotherapy helps general body movements and occupational therapy usually specifically targets hand function. Occasionally children make a good recovery and then develop difficulty in using the affected hand later; this can sometimes be helped by drug treatment or Botulinum toxin injection.

Most children affected by stroke speak as they did before, but occasionally speech therapy is needed. The majority go back into their previous school; it is worthwhile preparing the ground so that teachers know what to expect and most doctors are very happy to prepare an appropriate report. Occasionally children need extra help in school, either with physical challenges, e.g. dressing or in the playground, or with lessons and some of these will need a statement of educational needs.

Table one

Common associations with childhood stroke

Children with known illnesses
  - Sickle cell disease
  - Cardiac disease
  - Meningitis
  - Immune-deficiency

Previously well children
  - Chickenpox
  - Recurrent tonsilitis
  - Minor head trauma
  - Anaemia

Conditions which cause increased blood stickiness
  - Factor V Leiden
  - Prothrombin 20210
  - Increased platelets

Conditions which damage the blood vessel wall
  - High homocysteine levels

Abnormal lipids
  - Hypercholesterolaemia
  - High lipoprotein (a) levels

Table two

Reducing the risk of recurrence

- Balanced diet: five portions of fruit/vegetables/day
                  Fat- and salt-containing foods as treats

- More exercise, e.g. walking to school

- B vitamin supplements: folic acid, B6, B12,
  Low dose aspirin 1mg/kg/day

- Anti-coagulants for specific circumstances

15
The specific problems of younger stroke survivors

DONAL O'KELLY

The numbers

Stroke is this country's third biggest killer after cancer and heart disease, and the largest single cause of severe disability. It is commonly seen as an affliction of old age, yet it frequently strikes people in the prime of life, often for no known reason. In the UK, each year over 10,000 people of working age have a stroke – an average of nearly 200 every week. Over 1,000 sufferers are under the age of 30. Recovery can be slow, difficult and sometimes only partial. However, with the right attitude and support, especially in the early stages, dramatic improvements can be made in the quality of life for most stroke survivors. Complete recovery is often possible.

Different Strokes, a charity run by younger stroke sufferers for younger stroke sufferers, recognises the need for a wider choice of services for younger stroke survivors to help them return to a full life and an active role in their community. Stroke survivors have to learn everything from new, slowly moving and improving one day to the next, learning to talk, walk and live again. Different Strokes aims to provide throughout the UK:

- A regional network of exercise classes and swimming sessions (over 24 classes are up and running)

- Practical information packs to survivors

- Access to counselling services

- Benefits and rights information

- Advice and information on education, special training and work opportunities

- A quarterly newsletter to keep members in touch with each other

- Interactive website

The points raised in this section draw directly on Different Strokes' experiences of working with younger stroke survivors, who frequently complain that help currently available has been designed primarily to meet the requirements of older people. Different Strokes advocates a need for a wider choice of services designed for younger stroke survivors, to help them return to a full life and active role in their community.

While in no way wishing to minimise the impact of stroke on older people and their families, Different Strokes suggests that the needs of a 20-year-old stroke survivor will be quite different to those of someone aged 80, not least because the 20-year-old is faced not just by years but, hopefully, decades over which to recover from stroke and cope with its impact on family, education, work and social relationships. Rehabilitation, therefore, must be planned carefully and appropriately to maximise the potential of younger stroke survivors to return to independent living. Different Strokes believes that addressing the following issues would facilitate this process and at the same time contribute to reducing long term dependence on health and social services.

The anecdotal nature of some of these issues is acknowledged but, in the absence of formal research evidence on younger stroke patients, it is hoped it may generate discussion on the needs of this important, but often ignored, group of patients.

The wish list

At the first onset of stroke, we want to be believed. We have often heard examples of people being treated by health professionals who appear not to understand that stroke can affect young people, with symptoms ascribed to other conditions, from migraine to being drunk.

We want to be looked after by staff who understand our specific needs. Specialised stroke nurses on dedicated stroke units would be a good start.

Younger adults with stroke often report distress at being admitted to and cared for on elderly care wards. Greater consideration needs to be given to the appropriate setting and location for the care and early rehabilitation of younger stroke patients while in hospital.

We want staff to be aware of, and address, not only the physical effects of stroke but also its emotional, social and psychological impact. Consideration should be given to providing/improving access to counselling to help younger stroke survivors come to terms and deal with both the short-term effect of stroke but also help us adjust to its long-term implications for housing, personal finances, education and employment.

At discharge from hospital, we do not want to be 'written off' as disabled. We want a long-term plan of care which recognises that we are embarking on a slow but gradual recovery.

Existing discharge advice and information is designed to meet the needs of older people. Information on long-term care or nursing homes, for example, is usually not relevant to the needs of younger stroke survivors who want discharge advice tailored to their own specific short- and longer-term needs and circumstances. The bingo and basket-weaving currently available at the local day-centre is not always appropriate!

The goals of most younger stroke survivors include achieving, as far as possible, a gradual return to independent living, to employment and re-integration into family and social life. Those who design and provide services need to recognise that these goals may differ from those of older people and tailor rehabilitation services accordingly. Emphasis needs to be on treating the patients as individuals, taking age and personal factors into account.

After discharge, the transitional nature of recovery from stroke means that we should have an open-ended commitment to ongoing monitoring and assessment of our recovery so that rehabilitation services meet our needs appropriately as they change over time. This could be facilitated by ensuring that, as patients, we have details of a specific person who can be contacted to organise re-assessment of our needs as we progress in our recovery.

In meeting the goals of younger stroke survivors, rehabilitation services need to address the specific issues of re-education, retraining and re-employment.

Recognising that existing health and social services cannot meet the full range of ongoing and long-term rehabilitation needs of younger stroke survivors, consideration should be given to developing innovative ways of meeting some of these needs. Models such as GP schemes for prescribing exercise, opportunities for using leisure centres, etc. merit further investigation.

Younger stroke survivors have a range of information needs, including general advice on disability and help on getting aids and gadgets; information on benefits, social services and patients' rights; applying to charities for individual grants; coping with the psychological impact of stroke and people's attitudes to stroke; advice on sex and relationships (notes on these topics are produced by Different Strokes). NHS purchasers and providers should ensure that younger stroke survivors have timely access to these or comparable leaflets.

A number of organisations can provide advice on the specific issue of helping people with disabilities back to work. Health professionals in primary, community and secondary care need to be aware of the different organisations that can help younger stroke survivors, and need to convey this information to these younger survivors in systematic and timely ways.

Carers of people with stroke have their own support, advice and information needs. Special consideration needs to be given to address the needs of carers of younger stroke survivors, taking into account both the possible long-term nature of this caring role and its transitional and variable nature over time.

The hidden side of stroke

In younger people a stroke happens suddenly. It is a traumatic and devastating experience. We are somewhere in the course of our daily life when it strikes – at work, on holiday, relaxing at home, socialising with friends, or even asleep. Wherever we are, or whatever we are doing, our lives are brought to a complete standstill. Because many of us have had no previous experience of severe illness, the devastating effects of stroke are even more difficult to deal with. Stroke is about loss. The sudden loss of a fully functioning body and mind which we have always taken for granted. Now, instead, we have paralysed arms and legs, an inability to speak or be understood, incontinence, lack of concentration, poor vision, no short-term memory, uncontrollable laughter or tears, or any combination of the above and more. We find it very hard to relate to ourselves as 'ill' people, let alone disabled in some way.

Possibly, we have never been in hospital before, but almost certainly we will now experience hospitalisation and/or rehabilitation units, usually for weeks or even months. We are removed from life, work, relationships, friends and leisure time and become institutionalised as we begin the long, slow and difficult process of rehabilitation. Anyone who has had a stroke will know about the huge changes that it brings about. The loss of the freedom to 'get on with life' whilst the rest of the world goes by. We are not allowed to function as before but are left feeling vulnerable, helpless, without dignity, frightened and isolated.

141

This is the invisible side of stroke. No one can see those feelings, or those thoughts. Others can only see the sudden functional loss of parts of our body and, of course, it is vital that we work as hard as possible to regain as much as we can of what we have physically lost. However, it is equally vital that we allow ourselves to consider the 'invisible side of stroke'. It is not only our bodies which have been damaged, but our thoughts and feelings too. It is totally impossible to have a stroke and not experience extremes of emotion, fear and anxiety about life, work, family and close relationships, but most of all emotions about our relationship with, and perception of, ourselves. Everything changes after a stroke and everyone's recovery is individual. The most vital thing is that we give ourselves the very best chance of getting better.

It is not easy to ignore the physical changes which a stroke causes, but it is easy to ignore the 'invisible' ones. Acknowledging them and facing them can give us a fuller, more rounded recovery.

Different Strokes offers an opportunity to talk over the phone, or to meet with other stroke survivors at regular exercise classes. This will give you a chance to share your experiences with other people who have suffered similar loss themselves. It can help to remove the sense of isolation which having a stroke so often causes.

Ten years later Different Strokes reports: Donal O'Kelly has now moved on and lives in Ireland, but the organisation he founded goes from strength to strength, supporting groups scatttered throughout the UK. Different Strokes has successfully put young stroke patients high on the agenda.

Different Strokes: Telephone number: 08451 307172
Website: www.differentstrokes.co.uk
Email: different@strokes.demon.co.uk

Part 4

RESEARCH

16
An introduction to research

THE WHOLE OF THIS BOOK is some kind of crescendo – progressing from the mainly anecdotal via the advisory to the academic. The first part of the book does not include references, but the referenced content builds up in the next sections. Research is being undertaken at many different levels all round the world. This introduction gives the general reader an idea of some projects sponsored by charitable foundations in Great Britain.

The Stroke Association

The Stroke Association is the largest charity funder into stroke research in the UK, spending about £2.5 million on research projects alone each year.. From the extensive list of the projects it has funded in the past few years several have a direct bearing on subjects dealt with in this book, and just a few are listed:

Study of outcome of childhood stroke – Dr F O'Callaghan, Dr A Williams, Dr F Kirkham, Dr V Ganesan, Institute of Child Health, Bristol Royal Hospital for Children

Use of a metronome with variable beats to retrain walking in stroke survivors – Professor A Wing, Professor C Sackley and Dr D Pratt, University of Birmingham

A Very Early Rehabilitation Trial – UK – Professor P Langhorne,
   Dr O Wu, Professor A Ashburn, Professor Helen Rodgers,
   Dr J Bernhardt, University of Glasgow

*Reading in Aphasia: development of an assessment of reading
   comprehension* – Dr J Morris, Dr J Webster, Professor D Howard,
   Mrs J Giles, Dr A Gani, University of Newcastle

A full list of currently funded research project and programme
grants can be found on The Stroke Association website.

Other charities supporting stroke research

Chest Heart and Stroke Scotland
   www.chss.org.uk

Northern Ireland Chest Heart and Stroke
   www.nichsa.com

Connect – A charity set up for those with aphasia, a problem or
   disability in language and communication when communication
   centres in the brain are damaged often caused by stroke.
   www.ukconnect.org

Different strokes – A charity set up by stroke survivors to help stroke
   survivors of working age.
   www.differentstrokes.co.uk

Action Medical Research – A UK charity dedicated to helping and
   funding research for children and babies affected by disease and
   disability.
   www.action.org.uk

The next and final chapter, contributed by the team from
the Behavioural Brain Sciences Centre, the University of Birmingham, is based on work sponsored by the Stroke Association.
It explains how experimental psychologists organise and prepare
their research into cognitive rehabilitation.

17
Taking part in neurorehabilitation research

AMY ARNOLD, PARISA NASRI, TRUDY PELTON, ALAN WING
SYMON LAB (SCHOOL OF PSYCHOLOGY, UNIVERSITY OF
BIRMINGHAM)

'I jumped at the chance to help, when asked by a researcher at the SyMoN lab at University of Birmingham. I learnt to love getting out of the house again, widening my horizons. I loved talking to new people as I had only really been to rehab previously. I enjoy the challenge of the tasks because I am quite competitive but, more importantly, I want to continue to improve my movement ability.

I would very much recommend participating in research because not only does it help others in the long term, but being at the University is delightful – you're looked after so well and it's not time consuming because you are picked up and dropped home, no inconvenience. Good practice, great fun and increased knowledge.'

CATHERINE GOULD, regular participant in stroke research
at the University of Birmingham

This chapter aims to give the sense of what it means to take part in research into neurorehabilitation. We, the authors, are researchers studying the control of movement and disorders of movement following stroke. Here we talk about two projects which we are involved in to give the idea of the nature of research.

The participant experience:

Before any research participation can commence, participants are expected to sign a form to say they understand the nature of the research in which they are being asked to participate and that they are happy to be involved in the research. The consent form highlights that participation is 100% voluntary; participants may withdraw at any time and without giving a reason. The institution hosting the research will cover transport costs; and in most cases, participation won't take up more than a couple of hours of a participant's time in one visit.

Recent research example:

The most prevalent physical disability evident post-stroke is hemiparesis; muscle weakness in the upper and lower limbs of one side of the body (usually, the upper limb is more affected than the lower limb). In some cases all movement is lost on one side of the body which is called hemiplegia.

A recent study investigating whether the use of a metronome beat combined with arm and hand movement training enhances reaching and grasping in a stroke participant suffering from hemiparesis was carried out in the Sensory-Motor (SyMoN) Laboratory in the School of Psychology at the University of Birmingham.

Reach and grasp movements were specifically targeted for training because they can be particularly affected by stroke and thus, severely limit the ability to efficiently use the hands to carry out activities of daily living. Diedrichsen et al (2007) highlighted that coordination is a crucial part in successful motor control as the movement of one body segment, by one set of muscles, relies heavily on predicting the movement of a second body segment, moved by another set of muscles. For example, during reaching the hand opens to grasp the object, there is tight coordination between hand opening and reaching by the arm. The time to maximum opening (aperture) between the tips of the thumb and finger is linked to the timing of maximum speed of the hand towards the object. This implies that, in opening the hand, the brain predicts how the hand will approach the object.

Training co-ordination in reaching using a metronome beat:

Training combined with a rhythmic auditory beat was conducted over a period of two weeks. Participants were required to
reach, grasp and lift a target object in time with the beat. Each
movement consisted of six sub-movements, with each sub-
movement completed in time with one metronome beat as
follows (see Figure 1):

1. reaching and grasping the object from position A;
2. moving object to position B;
3. returning the hand to start button;
4. reaching and grasping object from position B;
5. moving object to position A;
6. return hand to start button.

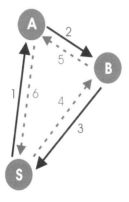

Figure 1. Diagram to show six sub-movements of the reach to grasp
(training) task. Black arrows illustrate first three movements (1–3), red,
dashed arrows highlight three, return movements (4–6). Distances between
position A, position B and start button (S) are to scale.

The sequence continues with the participant moving the object
between the alternate positions until a period of 40 seconds is
complete. The participant then rests for 20 seconds before the
next training trial begins. Each training session consisted of four

parts of 15 minutes of training, separated by 5 minute rest intervals. The interval between beats was matched to the participants' self-paced comfortable movement frequency, which was assessed in some initial baseline sessions. The metronome interval was progressively decreased by 5 to 10% each session, depending on the ability of the participant and experimenter judgement. For example the initial interval between beats for one participant was 1.7 seconds which progressed to an interval of 1.1 seconds in the final training session. Overall, training comprised approximately 9,840 movements, (of which 3,280 were reach to grasp) performed during six training sessions.

To determine whether training can improve reach and grasp coordination we used a special set of video cameras (Qualisys motion capture system) to track hand and arm movement during a task that involved reach, using thumb-index finger pincer grasp to lift a cylindrical object. Various features in the recorded data, including time taken to reach peak velocity (of the arm; i.e. the reaching component), movement onset time, maximum aperture (of the index finger and thumb; i.e. the grasping component), and total movement time were determined. The motion analysis took place on three occasions:

1. Before training (baseline measures)

2. Two days after training (post training measures)

3. One month after training (follow up measures).

In addition, the quality of the coordination between reach and grasp components was evaluated by asking participants to complete the tests at either a comfortable or a fast pace.

The findings from this pilot case study are promising. Data from a single right handed female aged 47 years with left cerebellar infarct suggest that when reach and grasp movement training is combined with a predictable, rhythmic beat, it significantly increases the temporal spatial stability (improved coordination) of hand and arm movements during reach to grasp movements. Also, it was found that training promoted increased speed and efficiency of individual components of reach and grasp at post training assessment; which was mostly maintained at follow up (one month after training ceased). For example, total movement duration decreased from baseline to post assessment (after training) and positive changes were still seen at follow up assessment for the comfortable pace, although it was not maintained at follow up for fast movements.

In summary, this study is providing insight into a promising strategy for upper limb therapy for stroke patients. The participants involved stated that the experience was 'challenging but enjoyable and beneficial'; with no negative side effects reported. Participants enjoy the time spent with researchers – discussing current research, findings, possible interventions for the future, sometimes just a chat about how the participant is feeling. Participants seem to relish the opportunity to talk to experts, and also Masters and PhD students recently commencing their research career.

Conclusion for the reach and grasp study:

The auditory metronome beat is a safe and cheap adjunct to upper limb rehabilitation which is easily incorporated into any clinical or home setting. The additional sensory cue appears to induce spatial and temporal stability for practised patterns of movement. Patients seem motivated by the beat to train the hemiparetic limb over and above their usual activity levels and beyond the training intensities often reported in the literature. It is with this increased intensity levels that we hope to induce behavioural change and to promote neural plasticity.

Psychology and Neurorehabilitation:

Stroke patient participation in research is vital to continuing to improve products and services available to enhance quality of life post stroke. Neuropsychologists dedicate their time to conducting research to enhance the understanding of the precise mechanisms underlying various aspects of behaviour, ranging from slow or weak movements in hemiparesis to cognitive deficits affecting attention and perception.

Cognitive deficits (e.g. attention, perception, language, memory) are harder to detect than hemiplegia, but no less vital to successfully completing activities of daily living (e.g. dressing, making dinner etc). Some cognitive deficits evident in stroke patients can affect learning and memory; for example, we were recently testing a participant involved in a study investigating the efficiency of reach and grasp movements after training post-stroke – the patient asked for a demonstration of the sequence of the arm and hand movements within the training as he was unable to remember from the previous session.

Neuroplasticity:

One of the most impressive features of the human brain is its ability to 'repair itself' following injury – a capability referred to as 'neuroplasticity'. Neuroplasticity refers to the area/s of the brain that were previously dedicated to one particular function but may take on additional functions, as injury will have diminished the function of these brain areas. Studies on the natural course of change following brain injury demonstrate that partial recovery of function does occur (Wilson, 1998). Brain scanning using functional magnetic resonance imaging (fMRI) provides evidence that there is increased activity in brain areas surrounding the lesion (Marshall et al, 2000). Much research suggests that motor behaviour of a certain level of intensity encourages neuroplasticity after neurological injury, so the level of physical recovery relies heavily on the experiences of the patient. Hence, it is of huge importance that stroke survivors continue to exercise and train the affected limbs.

The beauty of neuroplasticity is that it does not exclusively promote the recovery of physical deficits but also of cognitive impairments. Increasing evidence suggests that interventions (training, compensatory aids etc.) reduce the occurrence of cognitive deficits, and the extent to which these problems interfere with social and emotional functioning. Evidence of neuroplasticity provides a strong and encouraging platform for neuropsychologists to study new techniques and therapies. Growing understanding of such mechanisms has enabled new methods of rehabilitation for stroke survivors to be developed, which can significantly reduce both the frequency and duration of one-on-one treatment. However, all therapy or intervention suggestions need to be supported by scientific evidence of the mechanisms underlying these changes for new treatments to be widely adopted.

Research aims:

The motivation for conducting research investigating post-stroke deficits includes the following aims:

- **ACTION**: Gather a wide range of data on post-stroke cognition, physiology, neuroanatomy and behaviour.

  AIM: Increase current knowledge and deepen understanding.

- **ACTION**: Provide evidence to support innovative, effective and accessible rehabilitation interventions to increase successful rehabilitation outcome.

  AIM: Patients become increasingly able to carry out activities of daily living – improves quality of life, decreases the likelihood of depression.

Cogwatch – an exciting new multidisciplinary project led by UOB

Now that we have covered the process a researcher goes through when planning a study, we go back to tell you more about what participants are likely to experience. To do this, we introduce you to an exciting, new, innovative project called 'CogWatch'. The CogWatch project is based at the University of Birmingham and is funded by a grant from the EU.

The CogWatch project:

CogWatch focuses on patients with Apraxia and Action Disorganisation Syndrome (AADS) – see box below. The project aims to develop a new personal healthcare system for AADS patients, which is capable of delivering personalised rehabilitation at home.

What is AADS (Apraxia and Action Disorganisation Syndrome)?
Apraxia can be understood as an *"inability to perform skilled, sequential, purposeful movement" (Banich, 2004).*

Action Disorganisation Syndrome has been used to describe patients with *"selective impairments in carrying out multi-step everyday tasks, which are not linked to movement deficits" (Morady & Humphreys, 2009).*

So, Apraxia and Action Disorganisation Syndrome are disorders of learned movement. This means that everyday tasks such as making a cup of coffee, which were performed automatically before having a stroke, can no longer be performed efficiently. Although a patient's movements may be affected by their stroke, the impairments exhibited in everyday tasks by AADS patients are primarily cognitive, i.e., impairments in mental processes.

One way to understand this is to explore how everyday tasks are carried out by neurologically healthy adults. For example, in order to carry out an everyday task like making a bowl of cereal, an 'action plan' must be formulated. The action plan specifies the goal (making cereal) and the separate actions that enable the goal to be achieved (e.g., pour the milk, put the milk down). Importantly, the actions need to be organised into a sensible order; the cereal should be poured into the bowl before adding the milk. AADS patients have difficulty selecting and using the correct objects for the task and ordering the actions into an appropriate sequence.

> A patient's performance on an everyday task can be measured by the errors that they make. Patients with AADS most typically omit steps of a task (e.g., make cereal without milk) or sequence the steps of the task incorrectly (add sugar before cereal).

CogWatch aims to improve patients' independence:

Perhaps as many as 68% of stroke patients meet the criteria for AADS (BUCS, 2007). The difficulty these patients experience in sequencing everyday tasks means they are more dependent on caregivers and healthcare systems, and that they are frequently unable to live independently (Sunderland & Shinner, 2007). So, the socio-economic impact of AADS is huge. Although research has been carried out and therapeutic programmes have been devised to rehabilitate AADS, the principle focus has largely been on physiological rather than cognitive rehabilitation. Clearly, there is a need to provide effective rehabilitation. CogWatch aims to improve patients' independence by providing a personalised rehabilitation system that can be used at home and can provide long-term support.

CogWatch patient studies:

Patient studies will focus on helping patients with meal preparation, washing and dressing. In the early stages of research CogWatch aims to determine the types of feedback and cues that will enable patients to complete a task successfully. We aim to:

1. Guide patients through everyday tasks to prevent action errors.

2. When an action error does occur
   a. Make patients aware of the errors committed
   b. Make patients aware of the appropriate actions

By tracking the movements made by patients whilst performing

155

everyday tasks and by tracking the objects they use, we hope to develop a device that will be able to predict when a patient makes an error on a task. CogWatch will then be able to guide the patient towards successful completion of that task.

CogWatch in a patient's home:

The following scenario shows how CogWatch might be implemented in a patient's home.

A wearable CogWatch that provides feedback about the task, using images, sounds and vibration.

A Virtual Task Execution (VTE) module – a large screen, which can guide patients' actions by providing words or images of the task being undertaken. VTE synchronises virtual hand movements with real hand movements, by detecting position, so that CogWatch always knows which task is being carried out.

Participation in CogWatch experiments:

CogWatch will take approximately 3 years to develop. During that time, researchers at the University of Birmingham will be running many experiments. These will include assessing and classifying patients with AADS, exploring the effectiveness of different types of cues and feedback (see experiment below), as well as obtaining brain scans before and after rehabilitation, to enable researchers to explore whether changes have taken place in the brain. The participation of willing volunteers with AADS in these experiments is vital to the successful development of CogWatch. Participating in research is 100% voluntary and participants may withdraw at any time, without giving a reason. The institution hosting the research will cover transport costs and participants won't be asked to participate for more than two hours in any one visit.

CogWatch Case Study

Mrs AB is a patient with AADS (Apraxia and Action Disorganisation Syndrome) who has been assessed as someone who can benefit from using CogWatch. She has received training with CogWatch within a controlled hospital environment and now she is using CogWatch in her home.

Mrs AB is preparing breakfast by putting everything she needs on the countertop. She starts by taking a teacup out of the cupboard and placing it on the countertop. The CogWatch infers that Mrs AB wants to make a cup of tea and activates VTE to guide her through the task. Soon, VTE displays a representation of the items that are on the countertop including the cup, kettle, and tea caddy. It displays two virtual hands – a mirror position of Mrs

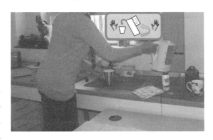

AB's hands. The hands on VTE move towards the virtual tea caddy. Mrs AB copies their action and moves towards the real tea caddy, takes out a teabag and puts it in the cup. She can follow this on the screen if she needs to.

Then she moves her hand towards the kettle (following the screen images) but instead of turning it on to boil the water she picks it up to pour the water into the cup. Cogwatch detects the error and activates the error recovery mode. As Mrs AB is in front of the VTE panels, CogWatch displays an error message that she can clearly read and a vibration from the wristband of CogWatch. The hands on the screen indicate the recovery by moving the virtual kettle back to its place and turning it on to boil the water. She boils the water and finishes making her tea.

Example of a CogWatch experiment at the University of Birmingham:

Aim: To guide patients through a cereal making task

Participants will sit at a table with all the equipment needed to make cereal (and some extra items – not related to toast making, but that can be used in the kitchen nonetheless – these are called distractors).

They will be asked to make a bowl of cereal with milk. Whilst they are making the cereal, participants will be videoed, so that researchers can understand the errors that they make on the task. The movement of their arm/hand will also be tracked by a motion capture system, which will allow researchers to understand the exact movements that patients are making. This will simply involve having several reflective markers attached to the skin.

Participants will then complete the cereal making task again, but this time they will receive 'visual cues' to guide them through the steps of the task. These cues will be photographs of the next action in the sequence. See below for an example of a sequence of visual cues.

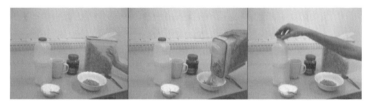

Figure 2. Pictorial cueing of steps in preparing cereal.

The participant will complete the cereal making task using the visual cues several times. The last time they repeat the task they will perform it without cues again, to see if there is any change in their performance compared to when they first completed the task. This helps to determine whether cueing has helped patients to learn the task.

> **How does 'cueing' work?**
> Providing step-by-step actions means that patients no longer have to use their impaired representations of the task in order to complete it, but can use the photographs as visual prompts, or cues for action.
>
> Additionally, research has indicated that observing specific movements performed by another person can prepare (prime) the sensorimotor system for subsequent motor practice (see Pomeroy et al. 2011). We propose that observing photographs of everyday actions can prompt the correct action or sequence of actions and therefore help people complete the task successfully.

What are the benefits of participating in CogWatch?

CogWatch is an extremely innovative research project which proposes a real response to the needs of patients with AADS. Participants who volunteer to take part in CogWatch will serve as a sample of patients, through which a global understanding of AADS will be developed.

The systematic and comprehensive assessments in CogWatch will enable participants to understand the nature of their difficulties and abilities more clearly. This will contribute to the development of a personal rehabilitation system which aims to improve patients' independence.

If participants stay in the project, it is hoped that they will see an improvement in their functioning on everyday tasks and will benefit from state of the art technology to further their rehabilitation.

Participating in research can be a rich and rewarding experience in which patients can meet and talk to experts about their illness, broaden their knowledge and experience of AADS.

Finally, CogWatch is a collaborative project and our strong links with the Stroke Association will improve general and public awareness and understanding of AADS.

Conclusion

Stroke patients with cognitive deficits report a decreased quality of life (Kwa, Limburg & deHaan, 1996; Riddoch, Humphreys & Bateman, 1995), and a higher incidence of depression. However, we can help! One research participant, Brin Helliwell, started to participate in research at the University of Birmingham a year after he suffered a stroke, listen to what he said recently...

"Being involved in stroke research has given me a positive out of a pretty negative situation in many ways. I benefitted hugely, psychologically, in terms of motivation and coming to understand what had happened to me."

Brin continues to involve himself in the research conducted at the Sensory-Motor Neuroscience (SyMoN) lab at the University of Birmingham and is regularly involved in charity bike rides and climbs to raise money for further stroke research. You can see a series of short films about how Brin got involved in research and its impact on his recovery at: http://www.crncc.nihr.ac.uk/about_us/stroke_research_network/patients_carers/index

Finally we would like to emphasise, that by participating in research, you may stumble across talents you've never previously discovered – or find techniques to enhance current hobbies. Take one lovely gentleman we tested a couple of months ago, a 64 year old who had begun to draw beautiful illustrations of his home town after losing most function in his dominant, preferred right hand post-stroke. He started to use his left hand to draw, supported by his right hand, and is now exhibiting his drawings over the county. See Figure 3 for an example of his lovely illustrations.

And it must be remembered that post-stroke improvements continue over one's lifespan – it is NEVER too late, you're never too old to get involved.

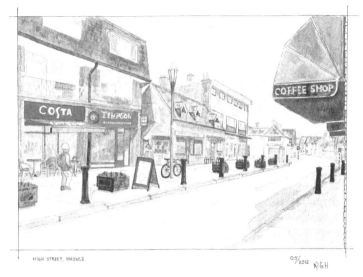

HIGH STREET, KMONLE.   05/2012 RGH

Figure 3. An example of a stroke participant's illustrations; he found a new talent in drawing after research participation at the UOB.

"Everyone has a 'risk muscle'. You keep it in shape by trying new things. If you don't, it atrophies. Make a point of using it."   ROGER VON OECH

The research process from a researchers' perspective:

Below is an overview of the research process (from a neuro-psychologist's perspective). We are leaving the scientific terms at the door so please do continue to read…

Identify a question your study aims to answer:
Does repetitive movement practice in time with a rhythmical beat encourage more efficient reach to grasp movements in participants post-stroke?

Design the way in which data will be collected:
Who is going to be tested? Age, gender, lesion location, nature and extent of deficit/s are all important characteristics to consider.
How often will the participant be tested and/or how many training sessions? It is common practice to employ a pre and post training

---

assessment. This enables the researcher to compare performance before and after training to see if their intervention is effective.

Write a research proposal for peers or sponsors to consider:
When looking for sponsorship or funding, researchers need to carefully and accurately outline the aims, design, predictions and clinical implications for their study. In other words, they need to provide a body of evidence that will help to persuade their 'investor' that their study is worthwhile and could dramatically and positively affect rehabilitation techniques used in the future.

Obtain ethical and trust approval:
Such approval is essential to ensure that the researcher's tests and training conform to the ethical principles embodied in the integrated research assessment system (IRAS; https://www.myresearchproject.org.uk/).
This protects the participants from taking part in research that might not be in their best interests.

Collect data with participants:
Have fun chatting with patients and discussing their experiences, informing them of the aims and predictions of the research whilst collecting data.

Statistically analyse data:
An integral aspect of any researcher's work – statistical analysis allows us to test whether improvements in performance from pre to post training assessments are reliable. However, it is important not to dismiss data that does not prove to be statistically significant, because trends within this data can still be observed and commented on and perhaps used to inspire further studies.

References

Banich, M T (2004). *Cognitive Neuroscience and Neuropsychology*, 2nd edition. Boston

BUCS (2007) The Birmingham University Cognitive Screen [online] available from <http://www.bucs.bham.ac.uk/main.php > [2 May 2012]

Diedrichsen, J, Criscimagna-Hemminger, S E, & Shadmehr, R (2007). Dissociating timing and coordination as functions of the cerebellum. *The Journal of neuroscience*, 27(23), 6291–6301. Society for Neuroscience.

Kwa, V I H , Limburg, M, & Haan, R J (1996). The role of cognitive impairment in the quality of life after ischaemic stroke. *Journal of neurology*, 243(8), 599–604. Springer.

Marshall, R S, Perera, G M, Lazar, R M, Krakauer, J W, Constantine, R C, & DeLaPaz, R L (2000). Evolution of cortical activation during recovery from corticospinal tract infarction. *Stroke*, 31(3), 656–661. Am Heart Assoc.

Morady, K, & Humphreys, G (2009). Comparing action disorganization syndrome and dual-task load on normal performance in everyday action tasks. *Neurocase*, 15(1), 1–12. Taylor & Francis.

Pomeroy, V, Aglioti, S M, Mark, V W, McFarland, D, Stinear, C, Wolf, S L, Corbetta, M, et al. (2011). Neurological Principles and Rehabilitation of Action Disorders Rehabilitation Interventions. *Neurorehabilitation and Neural Repair*, 25(5 suppl), 33S–43S. SAGE Publications.

Riddoch, M J, Humphreys, G W, & Bateman, A (1995). Stroke: Stroke Issues in Recovery and Rehabilitation. *Physiotherapy*, 81(11), 689–694. Elsevier.

Sunderland, A, & Shinner, C (2007). Ideomotor apraxia and functional ability. *Cortex*, 43(3), 359–367. Elsevier.

Wilson, B A (1998). Recovery of cognitive functions following nonprogressive brain injury. *Current Opinion in Neurobiology*, 8(2), 281–287. Elsevier.

Acknowledgement

We acknowledge funding from the Stroke Association and EU FPT ICT Healthcare programme in supporting the research described here.

Some final thoughts

PUTTING A BOOK TOGETHER takes quite a time. You start with an idea, get it down, think and struggle some more and it gradually changes. It gains a momentum of its own until by the time it is finished it bears little resemblance to the original outline. It is sometimes rather disconcerting for the publisher but that is the only way I can work.

Recovering from a stroke bears some similarities to creating a book. You start slowly, not knowing the final outcome. With luck and some hard work your whole attitude changes. I am glad that I wrote Part 1 nearly two years after my stroke. I could not write it now. I have moved on and no longer think the same way. It is not only that I have learned a lot from researching the subject so that other opinions would get in the way of my original observations, but I look forward not back. I no longer think of myself as disabled, certainly not in my own home – unless I see myself reflected in someone else's eyes or attitudes.

You can tell that I have written different parts of this book at different times. But where do you stop? With recovering from a stroke; probably never. But with a book; that is different. I keep hearing things that I want to discuss and share, but if I do not stop soon everything will be out of date before this is even published. Things are beginning to move in stroke care, attitudes are starting to change. I hope this book will add to the momentum.

APPENDIX
Information on the internet

THERE IS A GREAT DEAL of useful information, at all levels, to be found on the internet. Here are some useful websites from a list provided by the Stroke Association:

Stroke Association
e-mail: stroke@stroke.org.uk
website: www.stroke.org.uk

World Health Organisation
website: www.who.int/whr

Medical Monitor, aimed at both GPs and patients
website: www.healthinfocus.co.uk

Different Strokes
e-mail: different@strokes.demon.co.uk
website: www.differentstrokes.co.uk

Royal College of Physicians
website: www.rcplondon.ac.uk

British Brain and Spine Foundation
e-mail: info@bbsf.org.uk
website: www.bbsf.org.uk

British Aphasiology Society
website: www.bas.org.uk

Disability Net, for disability news and information
website: www.disabilitynet.co.uk

Disability-shop. sells disability and care products
website: www.disability-shop.co.uk

AbilityNet, a charity giving free advice on computer and web
use for people with disabilities
website: www.abilitynet.co.uk

Website bringing disability information into the
twenty-first century
website: www.4dp.com

Internet stroke support group
members.aol.com/scmmlm/main.html
Newsletter: members.aol.com/scmmlm/nl.htm

Sign on-line, Scottish Intercollegiate Guidelines a network for
information about care in Scotland
website: show.cee.hw.ac.uk/sign/home.html

Support Groups, information on groups for almost any illness
or condition
website: www.patient.co.uk

British Medical Acupuncture Society, BMAS
website: www.medical-acupuncture.co.uk

Disability Rights Commission
website: www.drc-gb.org

FOR CARERS

Developed by Action for Carers & Surrey County Council
website: www.carersnet.org.uk

Launched by the Department of Health
website: www.carers.gov.uk

Charity
    website: www.caring-matters.org.uk

FOR NURSES

Nurse Collaborative Group
    website: dcn.ed.ac.uk.ist3

FOR HEALTH CARE PROFESSIONALS

An information centre and forum, for the exchange of views with links to other strokesites
    website: www.strokeforum.com

British Association of Stroke Physicians
    e-mail: MSD@skull.dcn.ed.ac.uk

European Stroke Conference
    website: www.eurostroke.org

RESEARCH

Medical Research Council
    website: www.mrc.ac.uk

The MRC Brain Repair Centre, Cambridge
    website: www.brc.cam.ac.uk

Society for Research into Rehabilitation
    e-mail: ann.hughes@nottingham.ac.uk

BMJ (*British Medical Journal*)
    Full text of all information in editions of BMJ, available free on:
    website: www.bmj.com

INDEX

cramps 28–9, 40
crisis management 73–4
CT scans 132–3
cueing with CogWatch 158–9
Curtin University 67

Daily Telegraph article 22
darts 50
day centres 47
de la Mare, Ben 57, 61
dental checkups, importance 34
depression 24–5, 46
    countering 17–18
    in rehabilitation units 26
diet and nutrition in children 135
Different Strokes 51, 119, 128, 129,
    137–8, 142, 146
dignity 26–7
doctors
    junior 116–19
    see also GP
dressing 26–7, 155–6
drinking problems 27–8
driving 42, 67
drop foot 43, 65–6, 81–3
    bilateral 84
dropped foot stimulator, implanted
    84
dysarthria 94
dysphagia *see* swallowing problems
dysphonia 94
dyspraxia 94
dystonia 21, 29

eating problems 27–8
echocardiogram (ECHO) 133
educational needs for children with
    stroke 135
elbow extension 85–6
elderly people with stroke 129–30
electrocardiogram (ECG) 133
emoticons 62
emotional problems 101

in young adults with stroke 141–2
encouragement 68–9, 75
energy
    conservation 34–5
    utilising limited resources 41
    variations in 34
environment context 113
equipment *see* aids
exercise programme 67–9
    ARNI approach to functional
    recovery 105–15
    continuing 74
    with electrical stimulation 84
    for home 75
    repetition 113
    trainers 106, 108
    for young adults 137–8, 140
eye checkups, importance 34

Factor V Leiden tests 133, 134
family
    attitudes to recovery 42, 45–6
    role change 32
fatigue *see* tiredness
food charts 28
foot clumping 52
foot drop *see* drop foot
friends
    attitudes to recovery 33, 36–7, 42,
        45–6
    importance of 37
functional electrical stimulation
    (FES) 55, 66–7, 81–7, 90, 110
functional map expansion 112
functional recovery 71–2, 105–15

gadgets 40
    see also aids
gait
    analysis 66–7
    balance and 84
    problems 84
gardening 41, 55, 59, 60